Hope
Springs Eternal—
Surviving
a Chronic
Illness

Hope
Springs Eternal—
Surviving
a Chronic
Illness

David Atkinson

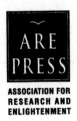

ASSOCIATION FOR
RESEARCH AND
ENLIGHTENMENT

A.R.E. Press • Virginia Beach • Virginia

Copyright © 1998
by David Atkinson

2nd Printing, December 2002

Printed in the U.S.A.

A.R.E. Press
215 67th Street
Virginia Beach, VA 23451-2061

Material on page 178 is from *The Public Perspective*, a publication of
the Roper Center for Public Opinion Research, University of Con-
necticut, Storrs. Reprinted by permission.

Library of Congress Cataloging-in-Publication Data
Atkinson, David R., 1935-
    Hope springs eternal : surviving a chronic illness / by David
R. Atkinson.
        p.   cm.
    Includes index.
    ISBN 0-87604-408-9
    1. Atkinson, David R., 1935—Health. 2. Amyotrophic lateral
sclerosis—Patients—United States—Biography. I. Title.
RC406.A24A85   1998
362.1'9683
[B]—DC21   98-10631

Disclaimer

The information in this book is not intended to replace medical advice.
You should consult your physician regarding any general or specific
physical symptoms. The author and publisher disclaim any responsibility for adverse effects resulting from information in this book.

Cover design by Richard Boyle

"The vast majority of patients diagnosed with various types of motor neuron diseases, whether it is ALS or other variations such as Spinobulbar Muscular Atrophy, do die within two to five years. Very few either stabilize or recover. David Atkinson's remarkable recovery should provide not only hope but a blueprint to be emulated with everyone with such diagnoses. His approach is safe, reasonable, and the only hope I know at this moment in time for these difficult diseases."

C. Norman Shealy, M.D., Ph.D.

Founder, Shealy Institute for Comprehensive Health Care

Founding President, American Holistic Medical Association

Research and Clinical Professor of Psychology, Forest Institute of Professional Psychology

"In his book *Hope Springs Eternal—Surviving a Chronic Illness*, David Atkinson has told his remarkable story of his healing journey through a devastating disease process. The book is truly inspired and any person who has the courage to face a disease in the way he has will certainly benefit from the healing program he followed."

Gladys Taylor McGarey, M.D., M.D. (H)

Founder, Scottsdale Holistic Medical Group

Foreword

This is the story of one man's transformation. Its message is relevant for all of us as individuals on a path of personal healing and to those of us in professions that promote healing in others. *Hope Springs Eternal—Surviving a Chronic Disease* is a deeply personal story with far-reaching lessons for all who read it.

Regardless of your position in the so-called health care revolution, you are undoubtedly aware that over the past fifty years (since Edgar Cayce's transition from this life in 1945) our system of delivering health care has changed dramatically. No longer are physicians the only recognized providers of the healing arts, and no longer are they the authority figures who dictate treatment to their childlike and submissive patients. Whether we are patients, clients, consumers—whatever term one uses—it is clear that the trend is toward collaboration between professionals and those they treat. (Members of the Search for God study groups will recognize this as Lesson One: Cooperation.)

The author of this book, my father, learned much on this journey about true healing of body, mind, and spirit—not simply symptom reduction. Professionals in the healing arts have much to glean from this work, this diary of transformation. We can learn the importance of listening to our hearts and inner voices, but, most important, to our patients and clients. It is time for providers of the healing arts and those we serve to work together as cocreators of wellness. By changing the orientation from treating or curing to *serving,* true healing can happen.

In *Hope Springs Eternal—Surviving a Chronic Disease* readers will learn of the author's personal program of self-healing (a redundant term, as all healing is self-healing). Described in deeply personal insights is his lifestyle change, including diet (he'd been a compulsive overeater for most of his adult life), his first explorations with meditation (a fad he previously attributed to hippies), a return to prayer (formerly seen as only for the weak and ignorant), as well as the painful attitude and thought-transformations that are at the core of any healing journey. Decades-old patterns of judgmentalism, criticism, selfishness, and negativity had to be carefully and painfully examined, accepted, and at least partially overcome.

While bookstores have been flooded in recent years with volumes promoting every conceivable method of "alternative" treatment, most are written by professionals based on their work in others' lives. Or they are written by individuals with advanced degrees or research grants or professional expertise. However, this diary of personal transformation is written by the one who experienced it. He has no degrees, no research grants, and prior to the beginning of this journey no experience in any healing arts. This story will touch you and may spark within you the urge to more closely examine your own life. The single most important statement in the volume will ring in your ears and heart long after you've finished reading it: *"When I said at the end of six months that nothing was happening, I had failed to notice that I was still alive!"*

Debbie Atkinson, M.S.W.
March 1998

1

What a beautiful day! The sky was a clear, bright blue—not a cloud in sight. The sun was warm and soothing as it caressed my body. I removed my shirt in order to improve my suntan and pushed the lawn mower through the tall, thick grass in our back yard.

My mind was racing almost as fast as the engine on the lawn mower. We would soon be off to Florida to start a new lifestyle in a fascinating and wondrous new place, and my thoughts were filled with excitement and anticipation. My wife, Wendy, and I had been planning this exciting family adventure for months. Every detail had been listed in our "adventure book" and studied thoroughly.

The entire family had been studying all the information that we had gathered about what soon would be our new home. Our seven-year-old daughter, Amanda, was proud of having memorized the state motto. She also knew the official state bird and could describe the flag in detail. We had spent many fun-filled evenings together as a family, planning our great adventure.

The moving truck had been reserved and scheduled. Wendy had given our former business partners her notice and was completing the final phase of training a new manager in the furniture store she had set up and managed from its conception. We had sold our interest in the store and in the furniture manufacturing company that I had started several years before. I had only one week left at the manufacturing plant.

We had disposed of our property, including a rental home, for a small profit, and I was due $9,000 from the company for back salary that had been deferred during a business expansion period. We were finally prepared to start our adventure.

Suddenly, the lawn mower engine abruptly stopped. I had run into a low spot in the yard where the grass was very thick, and the mower engine had stalled. I backed up several steps with the mower and reached down to pull the starter rope. As I leaned over, my head flopped forward, and my chin rested on my chest. It was as if I had lost control of the ability to hold my head up. A very strange feeling of weakness in my neck caused me to stand up without attempting to restart the lawn mower. As I stood there, my chin remained on my chest, and I realized that I was helpless to control the movement of my head. The sensation I felt in my neck was disturbing, so I decided to take a break and go into the house. I entered through the back door and immediately headed for the family room, where a beach towel hung over a wooden rack beside the fireplace. I grabbed the beach towel and laid it over the chair, and then I slumped down into the chair to rest.

The air conditioning was running, and the cool air felt good against my hot body. I laid my head against the soft back of the chair and rested for a while. After a short period of time my neck felt fine, and my hot, sweaty body cooled down. My head was back to its normal position. I went into the kitchen to get a drink of cold water, and everything seemed OK. It was time to return to the task of cutting the grass.

That day, my head flopped forward several more times before the grass cutting was completed and the lawn mower put away. As I came back into the house, my neck felt very weak, and my head was leaning in a forward motion, with my chin once again resting against my chest. Also, my swallowing seemed to be more difficult. Calling out to Wendy, I once again sat down in the family room to rest.

As Wendy entered the room, she commented about the position of my head. I explained what had happened while I was cutting the grass and that I had come into the house to rest, had returned to the yard, finished cutting the grass, and that now the problem seemed to be even worse than before. We both agreed that I should shower and give my body a chance to cool off and then lie down for a while and rest.

That evening, during dinner, I felt fine. As we ate, the conversation turned to what had become our favorite topic—our move to Florida. Wendy had received the school ratings for the area, just west of Jupiter Beach. This is where we had chosen to put down our new roots and start our new family adventure. We had made several trips to Florida and visited many different communities located in areas from the Panhandle to central Florida, as well as on the west coast and the east coast. We had decided on the Jupiter area because there was affordable housing, a good business climate, and fine schools and because my son David lived and worked in West Palm Beach, only about twenty-five minutes away.

After dinner, when Amanda was asleep in her room, Wendy and I watched TV until it was time for our evening exercises. We had both started on diets to become slim and trim as part of preparing for our new lifestyle. As I started my exercise routine by pulling down the grip bar, an exercise I had been doing regularly for weeks, my neck went weak again, and I couldn't keep my head from flopping forward. Wendy was doing her stretching exercises on the floor, when she looked up and saw what had happened to my head. Anxiously she said, "You need to see a doctor and find out what's wrong with your neck." The expression on her face showed her concern.

The next day I felt fine but agreed to call a doctor when I arrived at work. As I walked into my office, I was filled with excitement. This was my last week at work, and then we would have two more weeks left to complete our final moving preparations and to say goodbye to all our friends. My daydreaming was interrupted by the ringing of the telephone on my desk. It was Cindy in our sales department, checking on some items that had been placed on back order. I gave her the information she needed and asked her to bring all the new sales orders to my office. I wanted to complete the production schedule for the next five days.

There was a knock on my office door. It was Rick, my production foreman. We had our usual morning meeting. Then it was time for me to walk the production line, greeting each worker as I did every morning. There were no major problems that morning. Only two employees had failed to show up for work. I returned to my office to complete some paperwork.

The telephone rang again, and it was the receptionist. I had a call from one of my suppliers. He was confirming that the shipment of layered Dacron, the material we used to fill our cushions, was being shipped in two tractor-trailers and would arrive at our plant Wednesday afternoon. I checked the production schedule. Then I wrote a memo to the foreman of our sewing department.

It was my normal routine to visit the sewing department just before lunch each day to talk with Jimmy, the sewing foreman, and to say hello to all the ladies who worked in his department. Jimmy and Doretha were cutting fabric for a large umbrella order that was due to ship Tuesday. We spoke for a while, and I gave Jimmy the memo about the arrival of the Dacron on Wednesday. Then I spoke briefly with each of the ladies and returned to my office.

My telephone was ringing. It was Wendy. She wanted to know how I was feeling and if I had called the doctor. I explained that I was feeling fine, but she made me promise to call the doctor. We finished the conversation, and I wrote a note to myself to call the doctor after lunch.

One of my partners and I went to lunch at a local seafood restaurant, and when I returned to the office, I called the only doctor I could think of. It had been four or five months since I had visited his office during the flu season. After listening to me describe my symptoms, he said, "I think you should come in to the office this afternoon. We will work you in between 2:00 and 3:00." It was a surprise that he could see me so soon. Usually it took two weeks or more to get an appointment scheduled. "OK," I replied, "between 2:00 and 3:00 this afternoon." I finished some paperwork, talked to the production foreman and the sewing foreman, let the receptionist know where I was going, and headed off for my appointment.

The doctor asked a lot of questions. He looked in my mouth and down my throat and felt around my throat and neck. He placed his stethoscope on each side of my neck and listened, explaining that he was checking my carotid arteries. "I am unable to detect any problem," he said, "but I would recommend that you see a neurologist. Your symptoms might indicate some kind of neurological problem and that should be investigated immediately." He recommended someone he knew and said he would call and make an appointment for me. "No, thanks," I replied. "I'm going to wait and see if my neck bothers me again. If it does, I will follow up and see a neurologist."

2

Heading home, I felt great. It was a beautiful day, so I decided to surprise Wendy. When I arrived home early, she was on the telephone talking with someone at the furniture store. She finished the conversation and turned and gave me a hug. "Well," she said, "did you talk to the doctor?" I explained what the doctor had said after his examination. Then I took Wendy's hand and said, "Let's take a walk on the beach!" We lived five minutes from the ocean and often walked on the beach together. There was plenty of time for a walk because Amanda had gone home from school with her friend and we didn't have to pick her up for a couple of hours. Wendy didn't think that would leave enough time to get dinner ready, so I suggested that we get Chinese carryout after we picked up Amanda.

Off to the beach we went. We loved to walk along the beach hand in hand, enjoying the warmth of the golden sunlight, watching the gulls soar overhead, and listening to the melodious sound of the surf as it rolled up on the sand and then gently rolled back to the sea.

My mind was filled with many pleasant thoughts, some from the past but mostly thoughts about our life together in Florida. When we walked along the beach during the winter months, we had to bundle up with warm clothing, hats, and gloves. Sometimes the cold wind would slice right through our clothing, and the chill would reach my bones. In Florida we would be able to walk the beach together year-round with no heavy clothing and no bone-chilling wind.

I was so deep in thought that Wendy grasped my hand tightly. Evidently, she had been talking to me and realized that my mind was someplace else. "It's time to head back now," she said. I smiled at her. She was truly a dream come true for me, and I was fortunate to have found her. We turned and started back up the beach. I was thinking about our special song, which had meant a lot to both of us when we were dating—"I Like Dreaming," by Kenny Nolen. I planned to play that song on the stereo during dinner.

As we climbed the steps that led up from the beach, my head started to flop forward, and the weak feeling returned to my neck. Wendy was already at the top of the steps and turned to see what was slowing me down. When she saw my head, she rushed back to my side and took my arm. "Does it hurt? What can I do to help?" she asked. My speech was slightly garbled, and Wendy had difficulty understanding what I was saying. She grasped my arm firmly and helped me reach the top of the steps. "That's it!" she said. "You are going to see a neurologist and find out what's wrong, and you are going to do it first thing tomorrow morning!"

Dinner was not as I had planned it would be. I had some trouble swallowing and didn't eat very much Chinese food. I thought about putting our special record on the stereo, but my energy was so low that I just sat for a while in my favorite chair in the family room and rested.

Wendy got Amanda off to bed and then returned to the family room and sat down beside me on the arm of my chair. She was concerned. I could see it in her face as she said, "First thing in the morning, you are going to call the Plant and tell them you won't be in, because you are going to the doctor. Then you are going to go to a neurologist, and I am going with you! We must find out what is happening with your neck." I agreed and decided to go to bed early that night.

The next morning, I was up at my usual time, showered, got dressed, and had breakfast, but instead of leaving for work, I sat down in the living room and read over all the material that we had gathered about Florida. Wendy was getting Amanda ready for school. Amanda would get dressed and straighten up her room and make her bed. Wendy would help with any adjustments that were necessary. Then Wendy would pack Amanda's lunch for school, and they would both have breakfast together.

The living room caught the morning sun, and the rays of golden light seemed to dance through the large, French-style bay window. In the morning the living room was always a cheerful delight. It was a great room in which one could feel the flow of positive energy. My whole physical being felt as if it were being recharged.

Amanda came bouncing into the room. She certainly didn't need to be recharged! It was almost time for the school bus, and she threw her arms around my neck and gave me a big hug. Her smiling face seemed to fit right in with the aura of the glowing light that filled the living room. Wendy and I both walked Amanda to the front door. Two more hugs and she was on her way to the bus stop where the children gathered each morning to wait for their transportation to school. Wendy and I watched through the living room window until the children were on the bus and it was pulling away.

Wendy looked at me, and I knew what she was about to say, so I quickly said, "Dear, I'll call several friends who I know have had experiences with a neurologist and get some recommendations." First, I called the office and spoke with one of my two partners and explained that I would be in later on after I finished with the doctor. After a number of other calls and fairly lengthy conversations with friends regarding their medical experiences, one neurologist's name seemed to stand out. It was not the one that my doctor had recommended, but I decided to call for an appointment and explained what my doctor had said and gave the nurse a general overview of my symptoms. She put me on hold for a short period of time, then returned to the telephone. "The doctor's calendar is full for the next three weeks and—" I interrupted the nurse, "You see, I'm getting ready to leave town for Florida, and my doctor said, in his opinion, my condition could be something serious." The nurse asked me to hold on again. As I was waiting I thought maybe using the word *serious* would make a difference. When the nurse returned to the telephone, she indicated that she had discussed my symptoms with the doctor. If I wanted to come to the office and wait, the doctor would work me into the schedule. I thanked the nurse, got directions to the doctor's office, and told her, "I will be there in less than an hour." Wendy was supposed to go to the store that morning. There was no need for her to just sit there and wait with me, when she could be accomplishing many of the tasks that needed completing before we left town. When I explained my reasoning to her, Wendy agreed. So I left for the doctor's office alone.

As I sat in the doctor's waiting room, I found an interesting magazine article with some beautiful color pictures, detailing fish farming. "Maybe this is something that might work well in Florida," I thought. The article explained how the government was encouraging people to get into the business of fish farming and offered not only technical assistance but also financial help. I remembered that I had already put some information in a file that I had about fish farming.

Just as I was turning to the next page, a door opened and the nurse called my name. It was my turn to see the doctor. I was somewhat surprised, as the wait wasn't as long as I had anticipated.

The neurologist was about my height and in his early forties. After listening intently as I explained what had happened to my head and neck, he examined me and put me through several motion tests until my neck felt very weak and I could not hold my head upright.

The next day, I returned to his office for more tests and questions. He said, "Think very carefully about any and all changes or difficulties you've experienced physically in recent months." After several moments of thinking back over the past couple of months, I began to list the events that I could remember. "Well," I began, "I have experienced tightening of the muscles in the back of my neck and also in my right shoulder. As I remember back, there was some difficulty with my head movement at work, and I had been tiring more easily. And now I am having problems with my head flopping forward, a weak feeling in my neck, and also I have experienced some problem with chewing and swallowing food. Oh, yes, I have also lost my voice several times while speaking."

I wondered what the doctor would say about the new symptoms that I had mentioned. It's strange I hadn't remembered there being that many problems until the doctor asked me to think about them.

During this second visit, the doctor did more tests and a very thorough examination. He noted all my symptoms on his chart. His voice was pleasant, and his mannerisms were comforting. Whenever I had something to say, he would stop what he was doing, look me in the eye, and listen intensely. The examination was completed, and the doctor was writing as he sat at a small brown table and said, "These orders that I am writing are for you. You will need to take them with you to the outpatient lab at the hospital for some additional tests and blood work. My nurse will call the hospital and make all the arrangements. You are to be at the lab, which is located in the outpatient department, at 9:00 tomorrow morning. My nurse will call you when we have the test results from the hospital." I guess he could see the concern I was having by the expression on my face. "Next time when you come to the office, I'll have a better sense of what your symptoms indicate."

3

The next morning when I arrived at the hospital, it took me a while to find the outpatient department and the lab. I handed the papers that the doctor had given me to the nurse behind the counter. Wendy and I had both tried to read what the doctor had written, but neither of us could decipher much of the scratchy writing on the papers. The nurse said, "Have a seat and your name will be called when the technicians are ready for you. If you have to leave the waiting area to use the bathroom, make sure to check in again at the counter to see if your name has been called when you return." She reminded me of a first sergeant that I had known when I was going through military training. Her expression never changed, and her voice sounded like a recording.

I sat in the waiting area for about a half hour. When my name was called, I was led through a maze of corridors, traveling from one lab room to another. All in all, I was at the hospital for about two hours.

It was a relief to hear the young nurse's aide, who had been leading me around all morning, say, "Mr. Atkinson, you are finished with the test that your doctor ordered. You can leave now." I thanked her, made my way to the parking lot, located my car, and headed to the office.

It was about a fifteen-minute drive to the Plant, and I wasn't feeling that great, but there were things that needed to be done. There was only one day left at work to complete my obligations and bid farewell to my business associates and friends at the Plant. I had hired most of the employees, and after three years many of them had become friends. With all the exciting plans surrounding our move to Florida, I hadn't really thought about how much I would miss the business and the people that I worked with and cared about.

As I walked up the stairs to my office, I felt rather weak, so I went directly to my chair and sat down to rest. After a short period of time, I was back into my regular routine. As I left the plant that day, I was thinking that the next day would be the last day that I would drive this route from the Plant to home. As I looked in my rearview mirror, the sun was setting behind me, and I could see a bright orange glow. As I turned into my driveway and parked the car, my mind returned to the reality of my physical problems.

Wendy was busy doing things around the house, and Amanda was visiting with a retired couple who lived behind us. The conversation immediately turned to my hospital visit and the tests. My energy level was low, and I was feeling quite tired.

We sat in the family room and talked until we heard Amanda coming in the back door. She was smiling and, as usual, wanted to tell us both about what she had been doing. While Wendy finished preparing dinner, Amanda sat in my lap and gave all the details of her visit with our neighbors.

Wendy soon called to us from the kitchen, "It's time for chores. Dinner will be ready in ten minutes." It was Amanda's job to set the table. I usually served iced tea for Wendy and me, and milk for Amanda.

Dinner went slowly for me that night. I was having difficulty with my neck and head. My chewing was labored, and swallowing was causing me to continuously clear my throat. I didn't participate in much of the conversation. I left that up to Wendy and Amanda. I found myself leaning forward with my arms on the table. Even drinking my glass of iced tea had become a problem. "Dinner was great, dear," I managed to say, "but I'm going to leave the table. I'm not feeling very well." Amanda asked, "What's the matter, Daddy? Does your stomach ache?" I didn't know exactly what to say. I just tried to muster a smile. Wendy spoke up, "Daddy hasn't been feeling very well today. I think he needs to rest for a while."

As I sat in the family room, I could hear Amanda chattering away. She was so full of energy. I wished I could borrow some and energize my body.

An hour later it was time for Amanda's bath, and I was still sitting in the family room. Normally, I would be reading or watching television, but I felt uncomfortable. There were muscle spasms running down the back of my neck, and even though I was not eating or drinking anything, swallowing became more difficult than it had been before. I rested for a while longer and then decided to turn in early. I had hoped that the extra sleep would help me regain some additional energy.

I woke up early the next morning feeling good and ready for the big day. I showered, shaved, and got dressed. Wendy was awake, but the alarm hadn't gone off yet. I walked over to the bed, leaned over, and kissed her on the forehead. She smiled at me and started to get up, but I said, "Stay in bed. It's still early. I'm going to get breakfast on the way to work. You know, this is the big day. After all this time, I will be saying goodbye to everyone at the Plant." Wendy reached out and grasped my hand, "Have a good day, and don't overdo it." I squeezed her hand, waved, and walked out to the car.

As I drove to work, after having stopped for a traditional Southern breakfast of two eggs sunny-side-up, grits, sausage, sliced tomato, toast, and coffee, my mind was filled with thoughts from the early days when I first started my furniture business. Back then it was just me. I designed the furniture, constructed it, displayed it at a little shop I rented, waited on customers, sold the furniture, and then at the end of the day delivered it. The business had really come a long way in a short period of time. Wendy, who had been a regional controller with a large international retail chain located in England, took over the operation of our new retail store. The new business venture came together very well.

Then things started to change. Within the first four months, the decision was made to double the size of the new retail store. Phil and Robert, who were our partners, saw the need for the additional retail space, and Wendy and I agreed. Of course, this move required that more financial resources be put into the business.

Next came a change to our original marketing plans. We would expand our medium-sized coastal area to include the continental United States. Soon after, the Caribbean market opened, and we were shipping furniture to Puerto Rico. But Wendy and I felt that the business was expanding too fast. The expansion created additional debt, so even though business was good, we were not only reinvesting every dollar that came in but acquiring more debt.

It was at this point in time that I decided to concentrate on producing the product and leaving the financing and marketing to my partners. I had more than enough to keep me busy—hiring and training personnel, controlling inventory, buying new equipment, developing new designs, being responsible for production, and overseeing the packing and shipping department.

Suddenly, I was driving into the parking lot at the Plant. I had been so engrossed with my thoughts that I was unaware of the drive to work that morning. As I parked the car, I hesitated for several minutes so that I could clear my head and bring my thoughts back to the present.

As I walked up the stairs to the second floor, where the offices were located, my neck was bothering me a little, and my energy level was low. When I entered my office, there were some brightly colored packages on my desk and a pile of colored envelopes.

The rest of the day was spent opening goodbye gifts and cards and visiting with all my friends. The ladies in the cutting and sewing department had made some cookies and snacks. The day passed very quickly, and I bid my final farewell to all my friends and talked briefly with Phil and Robert. I knew that I would be seeing both of them again before I left town.

Wendy was at the store saying her goodbyes, and I stopped by on my way home to visit briefly with my friends there. Wendy greeted me as I entered the store. Her face beamed with that special, pleasant smile that always made me feel warm and tingly. I spoke with each of the ladies who worked at the store, hugging and exchanging best wishes. But by this time, I wasn't feeling very well. Most of my symptoms were returning, and my energy was just about depleted. I told Wendy about the way I was feeling. She suggested that I go home and rest while she completed some details at work. We walked together to my car and I drove home.

It took Wendy longer than she thought to complete the last-minute details at the store, so dinner was late. It was difficult for me to chew and swallow. Even though I felt hungry, it just wasn't worth the effort to eat. Wendy suggested that I have ice cream mixed with milk to help keep up my strength. The thought of going to bed without anything to eat was not very appealing to me, so I agreed to try a milkshake. Amanda's little voice joined into the conversation, "Mommy, can I have a milkshake with Daddy?" Wendy fixed us both a nice vanilla milkshake, and Amanda's face was beaming as she moved her chair closer to mine.

"Was today your last day at work, Daddy?" Amanda asked. "Yes, it was, Pumpkin." I often called her Pumpkin, and she had accepted the nickname readily. Wendy placed our milkshakes on the table. The tall dessert glasses were filled to the brim, and each had a colorful straw.

As I attempted my first sip of milkshake, the sudden shock of the cold temperature stopped me. Obviously, my throat was not reacting well to the cold temperature, but my taste buds were telling me that I wanted more. After explaining to Wendy what the problem was, she suggested warming the milkshake in the microwave. After several experiments, I ended up with a large glass of warm, thick milk. It was delicious, but I found that I had to drink very slowly because my head was leaning forward, with my chin almost against my chest.

Later that evening, I became aware that my head had fallen forward numerous times. Each time, I would raise it back to an upright position, just to find that it had fallen forward a few minutes later. That night was my worst, up to that point in time. I had trouble sleeping, even after taking my sleep medication, and my saliva caused more severe swallowing problems.

Saturday morning wasn't any better. The loss of sleep had exacerbated my physical problems. Wendy was very concerned and insisted on calling the neurologist to find out if there was anything we could do to alleviate my condition. When she called the doctor's number, she reached his answering service and was told that the doctor would be contacted as soon as possible and that he would call us back.

The telephone rang about forty-five minutes later. I was still in bed, where Wendy had been looking in on me every so often. As she came through the bedroom door, she had a strange look on her face. "The doctor wants me to drive you to the outpatient clinic at the hospital," she said. "He will meet us there. He said this would be a good time for him to do a special test, while you are experiencing these symptoms." I agreed to go, hoping he could tell me what to do or perhaps give me a prescription that would alleviate some of the problems.

Amanda had already been in and said good morning to me. Then she was off to a friend's house just down the block. Wendy called the parents of Amanda's friend and explained the situation and that we would be out for a couple of hours. Then she helped me get dressed and out to the car.

Soon we were pulling into the parking lot at the hospital. As we walked to the outpatient clinic, I had great difficulty holding my head up. Wendy took hold of my arm. "Don't worry," she said. "We will be there in just a moment." I tried to turn and smile, but we were already at the door. As we stepped onto the black rubber pad, the large double doors swung open and in we went.

The doctor was waiting, as he had promised. He came over to where we were and introduced himself to Wendy and then shook hands with me. "Follow me, please," he directed. We followed him down a hallway and into a small room. There were an examining table, numerous types of electronic equipment, several chairs, and a white curtain that slid along a metal track on the ceiling. The doctor indicated where Wendy should sit, and then he turned to me and said, "Take your shirt, pants, shoes, and socks off, then please get up on the examining table, lying on your back with your head at this end." He pointed with his hand to the end of the table that was closest to the wall.

He explained that he would be attaching a number of electrodes to different areas of my body, starting with my right side and including my head. "These are electrical conduction tests," he explained, "and you will feel some discomfort from time to time but nothing that will actually cause you any severe pain."

As I lay on the examining table for over an hour, attached to all those electrodes, my mind was spinning with questions. I had thought the doctor would give me a regular checkup or examination. I certainly had not anticipated all of this! I was experiencing muscle spasms, and the back of my neck was as stiff as a piece of pipe. Also, my swallowing was very labored. The doctor was using some kind of electric probe, and as he touched each location on my body, I could hear a loud scratching sound coming from the equipment. Suddenly, the lights went off on the electronic equipment, and the doctor removed the electrodes from my body. He helped me up from the examining table and waited as I dressed.

We all went into another smaller room where Wendy and I waited as the doctor folded paper tapes from the testing equipment and organized them in a large red folder. When he looked up at me, he said, "I have already seen the results of most of your lab work, and I need a chance to study the results of the tests that we just completed." At this point, I interrupted, "Doctor, what is going on? We are moving to Florida in two weeks. I need to get a prescription and get this problem cleared up!" I looked over at Wendy, who was staring intensely at the doctor. I wanted to say more, but my mind was so jumbled up that no words came out. The doctor put the red folder in his black bag, then said, "I would like both you and Mrs. Atkinson to come to my office at 8:30 Monday morning. I really don't have any firm answers for you at this time, but on Monday I believe that I will be able to explain to you both what you are experiencing and how we should proceed."

4

A light rain was falling as Wendy and I arrived at the neurologist's office on Monday morning. Not only was I experiencing more of my usual symptoms but I also had a bad headache and was feeling nervous and very apprehensive. Wendy had been trying to cheer me up and to lift my spirits, but I could see that she was nervous, as well.

The nurse led us down the short hallway to an office. The doctor was seated in a large, brown leather chair. As we were escorted into the office, he rose to his feet, smiled, shook hands with Wendy and me and said, "Please, have a seat." There was a single chair and a small couch in the office. Wendy and I decided to sit together on the couch. The doctor returned to his chair.

As he started to explain about what my symptoms and tests indicated, his voice became very soft, yet serious in tone. His face portrayed a slight reddish flush. The news was not good. His diagnosis was that I had most likely

developed a disease known as amyotrophic lateral sclerosis, ALS, also known as Lou Gehrig's disease. He explained it would be necessary for me to have a nerve and
muscle biopsy as additional confirmation of the disease.
Arrangements would be made for me to go to the University of North Carolina Hospital in Chapel Hill. He
knew a doctor there who was a specialist in neuromuscular diseases and particularly familiar with ALS, and he
wanted this doctor to do the biopsies. I could see from
his demeanor that he had a great deal of faith in the ability of this particular physician, so I agreed with his recommendation.

"I will explain, as best as I can, how this disease develops and its progression," the doctor continued. "The
cause of ALS is unknown. Certain brain cells die, and the
nerves that are controlled by those brain cells stop functioning. This, in turn, causes muscles to atrophy, or
waste away. As the muscles atrophy, or become weak,
they stop functioning, and those areas of the body where
the muscles stop functioning become paralyzed. In your
case, the first area to show signs of muscle weakness is
your throat and neck area. This is known as bulbar onset. If your arms or legs had been affected first, then it
would be known as limb onset. This is a very serious illness."

He handed me some literature that had been lying on
his desk and said, "This material will explain what can
be expected as this disease progresses. I know that both
of you have many questions to ask, but please take the
material home. Read over it together."

The doctor asked us to return to his office the next
morning at 11:00. He promised to do his best to answer
our questions and said he would schedule an appointment for our visit to Chapel Hill for the biopsies. As we
all stood up, the doctor put his hand on my shoulder and
looked directly into my eyes. I didn't see a sad expres-

sion on his face; rather, I saw a caring and concerned person. At that moment he was a friend, not just my doctor.

Wendy and I left and made our way to the parking lot, which was located behind the doctor's office. We both sat in the car and started to read through the material that the doctor had given us. As we read the words, I became very cold. My whole body seemed to be numb, as my brain absorbed the information that I read: "ALS was first identified in 1869 by the noted French neurologist Jean Martin Charcot. The cause, the means of control, or the cure for ALS is presently unknown. The onset of ALS is insidious, with muscle weakness or stiffness as an early symptom. Inevitable progression of wasting and paralysis of the muscles of the limbs and trunk, as well as those that control vital functions such as speech, swallowing, and respiration, follows.

"Mental faculties are not affected. Also, ALS is not contagious and is a disease which occurs throughout the world, with no racial, ethnic, or socioeconomic boundaries. It can strike anyone.

"Because ALS destroys certain elements in the nervous system, while sparing others, consideration as to its cause has been [confined] to agents with selected properties. These have included viral infections, toxic agents, and genetic factors. Approximately ten percent of ALS is familial, occurring more than once in a family lineage.

"Treatment is aimed at symptomatic relief, prevention of complications, and maintenance of a patient who is alert but functionally quadriplegic, with intact sensory function, bedridden, and aware he or she is terminally ill and dying.

"The financial cost to the victim and the families of persons with ALS is exceedingly high. Entire savings of patients are quickly depleted because of the extraordinary cost involved in the care of ALS patients." We sat in silence, stunned. How could something like this be happening to me! The silence was broken by the sound of a car engine starting up in the lot next to us.

I don't remember anything about the trip home except that Wendy drove. My mind was spinning. When Wendy and I spoke again, we were sitting in our family room. I felt very strange and uncomfortable.

Our family room was a very special room that held many memories of joy and happiness. When we entertained Amanda's little friends in that room, it was decorated with red, green, and yellow streamers and lots of brightly colored balloons. It echoed with laughter and squeals of delight as birthday presents were opened and games were played and candles blown out atop so many beautiful birthday cakes.

Wendy and I had some great family get-togethers with my older children, from my first marriage, and we always seemed to gravitate to the family room. During my first marriage, which lasted for approximately twenty years, there were four children—Deborah, the eldest, then Michael, David, and Pamela.

My first wife and I had married when we were both very young. She was eighteen, and I was nineteen. I was attending the University of Miami in Coral Gables, Florida. We were both away from home and our families for the first time, and we enjoyed each other's company. In fact, we were married within ninety days of our first date. She was from a rural area of North Carolina, and I had grown up in Washington, D.C. As our older children left home for school and marriage and started their own families, we realized that we didn't have very much in common and were not fulfilling each other's needs or growing and expanding our individual lives.

We had an amicable divorce with no unpleasantness; in fact, we were both very much relieved. My ex-wife took custody of our youngest daughter, Pamela, and I took custody of our youngest son, David.

I remained close to my first wife's family. In fact, when Wendy and I decided to get married, I took Wendy to meet them; and after Amanda was born, my first wife baby-sat for Wendy and me on a number of occasions, and Amanda has continued to visit with her over the years. Wendy got along well with my older children, and Amanda calls them her brothers and sisters. They all call her sister.

All of a sudden, I realized that my mind had been wandering. Now as I looked around the family room that had always been filled with joy, it seemed different. The bricks forming the fireplace looked cold and foreboding. The paneled walls seemed dark, almost sinister in nature. The room seemed smaller, almost foreign to me. As my eyes traveled from the ceiling fan to the floor, I suddenly realized that Wendy was sitting next to me on the couch. I turned and saw her face. She was looking at me, and as our eyes met, she took my hand and said, in a gentle, loving voice, "We need to talk before Amanda arrives home from school."

As we started to talk, it was obvious that we were both rambling. Neither of us knew what to say. There were many questions but very few answers. In fact, we had no answers. What were we going to do about our move to Florida? How fast was my illness going to progress? How do I tell the children, especially our seven-year-old, Amanda? We were both feeling anxious, and my emotional level was just about to overflow. I could feel the tears starting to well up in my eyes!

Hiss. We heard the loud air brakes from Amanda's school bus as it stopped in front of our house. Quickly, we decided to set the matter aside and talk about it later. Holding back my tears, I told Wendy that we would greet Amanda as if everything were normal. We heard the front door open, and in she bounced, full of energy, her face beaming with a beautiful smile and all excited about her day at school. She gave us each a hug and then proceeded to unleash her usual stories about what had happened that day at school. Her sweet, little voice darted excitedly from one story to another, almost without taking a breath.

I heard some of what she was saying, but my mind was churning. It was almost as if I weren't there with Amanda and Wendy. I could see them and I could hear them, but I felt removed, almost as if they were on a movie screen and I was seated in the audience. All of a sudden, I heard voices coming from the kitchen. It was then that I realized I was sitting on the couch alone and Amanda and Wendy were in the kitchen. Wendy was asking, "Did you eat all of your lunch today?" "Oh, yes, Mommy, I ate everything." The sound of her little voice penetrated the façade that I was using to stay calm.

I could feel my emotions building up again. I tried to relax by taking deep breaths and leaning my head back against the couch. Once again there was stiffness in my neck and spasms in my shoulder and throat. My mind was spinning, as my thoughts seemed to be crashing into one another. Nothing seemed to make sense to me! There were thoughts of Florida. I could see the beautiful shades of green among the tropical plants and colorful flowers, and the deep blue sea. Now other thoughts were invading my mind. How long did I have to live? Would I waste away slowly and in pain? What would Wendy and Amanda do? So much misery! What about my older children? How would this affect their lives? Was I really going to die? How could this be happening to me? Tears started to roll down my checks. I had lost control of my emotions. I felt overwhelmed.

How can I let Amanda see me in this condition! I got Wendy's attention and told her about what was going on in my mind. She took my hand and looked into my teary eyes, saying, "You need to rest. I'll tell Amanda that you have a headache and are going to the bedroom to lie down for a while." Wendy kissed a few of my tears away and motioned for me to go to the bedroom. I whispered to her, "I'm going to take a couple of sleeping pills and try to shut down my mind." She nodded her head yes, and I went to our bedroom. Wendy returned to the kitchen to help Amanda with her after-school snack.

Because I suffered from insomnia, I had been using sleeping pills for seven years. At first, I used them occasionally, but over the years, my use became more frequent and required higher doses as time passed by.

As I entered the bedroom, I closed the door behind me. My head was whirling with so many thoughts that I actually thought my head was swelling. I made my way to the medicine cabinet in our bathroom and stared into the mirror. My image was different than it had ever been before. My face was pale, almost chalk white. I quickly opened the medicine cabinet, reached for my medication, popped it into my mouth, and washed it down with a small cup of water.

When I closed the cabinet, once again I saw my image in the mirror. My eyes flooded with tears. Immediately, I turned away from the mirror, moved quickly over to the bed, and sat down to remove my shoes. I was exhausted and filled with anxiety. My mind conjured up the image of my face that I had just seen in the mirror. Suddenly, I was filled with fear. There was a feeling of being all alone, almost isolated. I quickly undressed, got into bed, and pulled the covers up around me.

5

Emotions—what could I do about my emotions? I was losing control. Crying and becoming fearful were only making things worse. I had never been an emotional person; in fact, I had always been proud that I could be calm and cool during stressful situations.

Starting in my senior year in high school, I belonged to a voluntary emergency ambulance service. When I went to the University of Miami, in Florida, I had a part-time job with a large ambulance company that handled all the emergency service for the city of Miami and Miami Beach. I became certified by the American Red Cross as a first aid instructor and assumed the duties of training officer for all emergency personnel.

Automobile accidents, stabbings, shootings, heart attacks, strokes, drownings, burn victims—every imaginable emergency or catastrophe one could think of were part of my daily routine.

I was a hands-on medic and took the lead in most serious situations. I had scores of people die in my arms. Many times my efforts were not enough to make the difference between life and death. But I helped save the lives of many more than I lost. The experience of the first baby that I delivered is forever etched in my mind. I delivered more than three dozen babies, including twins and several breech babies, during my time as an ambulance medic. And now I was in bed, bundled up under the covers, crying and scared. I did some deep breathing and tried to relax my mind and my body. I had calmed down considerably as I faded off to sleep.

The alarm sounded, and I sat up in bed with a startled feeling. Wendy reached over and shut off the alarm. I realized that it was Tuesday morning and that I had slept through Monday afternoon and night! Wendy and I kissed and held each other closely. She had a warm and loving expression on her face and whispered, "We'll have a nice breakfast on the patio."

After Wendy got Amanda ready and off to school, she prepared poached eggs—my favorite. We tried to make it a special occasion whenever we ate on the patio. We could see and smell the flowers in our garden, made all the more eloquent by the golden rays of the sun.

Even though I was already experiencing neck and swallowing problems, we had a relaxing breakfast that morning. My wonderful Wendy—she always made me feel loved. Our romance had been a wondrous, passionate love affair from the very beginning. We had never known love and passion that strong; at times it seemed that we had become one being.

During breakfast, I left most of my toast on my plate because of my swallowing problem. By lunch time, I was having difficulty holding my head upright, and as I chewed my tuna fish sandwich, it became more difficult to swallow and a real labor to continue chewing. I ate very little of my sandwich but did finish my iced tea.

The couch in the family room was my next stop. My head was flopping forward, my neck was so stiff that the muscles were experiencing severe spasms, and my throat felt as if it were closing. My speech was labored, and so was my breathing as I tried to clear my throat. My apprehension was growing stronger, and an ominous feeling gripped me. I was, once again, experiencing fear. I called to Wendy, who was in the kitchen, "Please come and help me. I'm having trouble breathing." She rushed into the family room and asked, "What's wrong with your breathing?" She knelt on the floor next to the couch. I looked at her and in a low whispering voice said, "I'm feeling very strange and am having difficulty with my breathing." I didn't tell her about my feeling of fear, which at this point was closer to a feeling of panic.

Wendy quickly helped me back to our bedroom, and I found a reasonably comfortable position with my chin tucked, lying on my right side. It seemed that I was producing an excessive amount of saliva and couldn't swallow easily. Wendy was sitting on the edge of the bed and touching my arm with a gentle, comforting motion. My voice was weak as I said, "Please, get a towel!" She understood what I had said and brought a rose-colored bath towel, which she placed on the bed under the right side of my face and chin. The saliva drained from the side of my mouth and onto the towel. This arrangement reduced my swallowing problem, and my throat relaxed enough that my breathing returned to normal. I calmed down and only at that point realized how scared I had really been. Fear was a foreign feeling for me, but I had actually been scared. More precisely, I had been frightened that I might choke and be unable to breathe.

My skin felt clammy, and my energy level was very low, but at least the fear had passed. I was much more relaxed physically, but now my mind had started to race. It was almost like watching a videotape over and over again. My emotions started to rise again, and my eyes became teary. It had to stop. I had to get control of my mind. Suddenly, a series of very strong muscle spasms jolted down my neck and into my right shoulder. The fear was starting to return to the point of panic. I asked Wendy to get me two sleeping pills and a cup of water. I tried several times to wash the pills down my throat. The water was coming out through my nose. Wendy told me, "Lie still for just a moment," and rushed out of the room. She returned quickly with a flexible paper straw. I was able, using the straw, to drink enough water to swallow my sleeping pills.

I grabbed Wendy's arm. My voice was very weak, and she had to lean forward to understand what I was saying. I begged her not to leave me while I slept, just in case I should start to choke. She said, "I will watch over you, dear." She was smiling as she looked into my eyes. I could go to sleep feeling safe.

When I woke up around 7:00 p.m., Wendy was just coming into the bedroom. She saw that my eyes were open and walked over to the bed. While I was sleeping, she had called the doctor and rescheduled our appointment time for early Wednesday morning. Our minds had been so overwhelmed that we both had forgotten that we were supposed to be at the doctor's office at 11:00 a.m. after our patio breakfast.

I couldn't eat dinner and had difficulty even drinking iced tea. But by using a straw, I was able to drink two glasses of milk. I was starting to worry more about my family, especially Wendy and Amanda. So many questions and no answers—I was becoming stressed out. Eager for Wednesday morning to arrive, I took another dose of my sleeping pills and returned to bed. It was the only way I knew to shut down my racing mind and the emotional roller coaster I was on.

Wednesday morning at 8:00 a.m., Wendy and I were

sitting in the doctor's waiting room. Despite all of the extra sleep that I had, I felt exhausted. Even though I was slumped over in the chair, supporting my head with my hand, my neck still felt very weak, and my head movement was difficult to control.

As I looked up, I saw the doctor walking toward us. He had a pleasant look on his face, and he took my arm to steady me as I stood up. He had a reassuring air about him, which created a calming effect over me.

The doctor listened intently as I described the events I had experienced. He made a few notes and then examined my neck. He used his little pen light to look into my mouth and throat. He felt around my jaw, chin, and down the front of my neck. He observed the spasms that ran down the back of my neck, into my right shoulder, and around the area of my Adam's apple. He also examined my eyes, arms, legs, and feet. He spent considerable time watching my face and neck area, as well as my right arm. So I asked, "What are you looking for?" The doctor pointed to a number of locations along my right arm and asked, "Can you see those little ripples of skin as they move down your arm?" I nodded my head yes. It was strange. I could not feel them, but I could see them quite easily. The doctor said, "Those are fasciculations, and you also have them in your neck area, as well as your tongue. They are to be expected with your illness. Also, when I looked into your mouth, your palate had no movement, and there were signs of paralysis around a small area to the right of your upper lip."

The doctor looked at Wendy and then at me. His voice lowered in tone as he said, "I am sure you and your wife have read the material about ALS that I gave to you. There is really nothing that I can tell you that wasn't covered in the written material. There is no known medical treatment for ALS, and you can expect your symptoms to continue to develop."

All of my symptoms, all the strange things that were happening, were to be expected, according to the doctor. I asked, "Isn't there anything that can be done?" and he shook his head from side to side and said, "No." Then he quickly added, "I think I can alleviate some of your problem, regarding holding your head erect and taking some of the pressure off your neck." As he reached for his prescription pad, he said, "I'm going to prescribe a soft neck collar for you." I was surprised and exclaimed, "A neck collar! You mean the kind that you see people wearing who have been in auto accidents?" "Yes," he answered, "I believe it will give you some relief."

As Wendy and I were leaving, the doctor said, "Try not to fatigue yourself in any way. No exercise, no alcohol, and try some very soft foods that don't require very much chewing." I then realized I had forgotten to tell the doctor how much difficulty I had swallowing water. I told him about my problem with water and how it had come out through my nose while I tried to drink it from a cup. He explained that, because my palate was not functioning, there was nothing to stop the water from entering my nasal cavity. He added that having difficulty swallowing water is another symptom of ALS. Thin liquids are the most difficult to swallow, but he told me about a product called Thick-it. One mixes it into a glass of water, making it easier to drink. He made another appointment for me to see him again in one week and said, "Don't hesitate to call me if there are any serious problems that might occur."

We took the prescription for the neck collar to a hospital supply store, just around the corner from the doctor's office. After trying several collars, I found one that seemed to work very well for me, and it felt comfortable.

As Wendy and I drove home, the doctor's words kept echoing in my mind: "Don't hesitate to call me if there are any serious problems that might occur."

Wendy and I had discussed, in great detail, our move to Florida and had decided the only choice we had was to put our plans on hold until we knew more about what was happening to me. This would mean cancelling the moving truck, making arrangements to stay on in the house for an extra two or three weeks, contacting the utility companies, and rearranging many additional details. Wendy told me not to worry about any of these problems. She would take care of everything. Of course I couldn't help being concerned, but it was reassuring to know that Wendy had everything under control.

Amanda was very disappointed and asked many questions that we couldn't answer. So we told her that I wasn't feeling well enough to take such a long trip right now. Of course this meant that Amanda would be staying in her present school until we figured out what we were going to do. Our original plan was to have Amanda start her new school in Florida even though the school year was almost over. We thought it would be a good way for her to meet a lot of the children in our new neighborhood and also become comfortable with her new school.

My condition worsened in general, especially my eating and swallowing. I could not chew or swallow any solid food, and I was losing weight rapidly. At my next appointment, the doctor gave me a prescription for a liquid nutritional drink called Ensure. He said that many people, especially ALS patients, lived on this special drink without any solid food in their diets. He was concerned about my weight loss and instructed me to make sure that I consumed at least 2,500 calories per day. I was to weigh myself every other day and call him if I continued to lose weight. As he was giving me the instructions about my diet, he looked at Wendy several times. I guessed he wanted to make sure she knew that my weight loss was a serious problem and that it needed to be turned around.

6

One evening while I was watching the news on TV, the phone rang. Wendy and Amanda were doing most of the telephone answering, because my voice had become very nasal in tone, and the more I talked, the more problem I had with my throat. My voice often gave out completely, right in the middle of a conversation.

Wendy answered the telephone. Something caused me to look up. Her face was flushed and her usual smile was gone. She was just standing there staring at me. Then she spoke, "It's David, Jr." David was my youngest son. Either I called him or he called me almost every week from Florida, where he lived and practiced law, but I knew he had been out of the country on business, so I hadn't heard from him for several weeks.

We had decided not to tell any of my children or anyone else, for that matter, about my health condition until we knew more about my situation. I took the phone from Wendy and tried a strong hello and asked what he had been doing. It was good to hear his voice, and he proceeded to bring me up to date on his activities. We had a good conversation, during which he commented about my voice. I laughed it off and told him I was just getting over a bad sore throat. Everything was going great, and I felt that I could make it through the conversation without alarming David. That would give me at least another week to figure out what to tell my four older children, who were all young adults living in different areas of the country. My oldest daughter, Debbie, had just moved to a new job in Salisbury, North Carolina. Debbie had worked her way through school as a divorced single parent with two small children. She had done her undergraduate work at Appalachian State University in Boone, North Carolina, and then completed her master's degree in social work at UNC, Chapel Hill. She had worked very hard, sometimes two jobs at a time. She was a good, loving mother, and her children were happy and well taken care of. The fact that she had been able to complete her education, along with all her other responsibilities, was a remarkable achievement.

David was saying, "Dad, are you still there? Can you hear me?" My mind had been wandering again. I made some kind of excuse about the telephone connection and said, "I can hear you fine now." Everything was under control, and I wanted to finish up the conversation as soon as possible. But then David asked about our timetable for moving. He said, "I thought you were due to be here in Florida by the end of this week?" My voice broke, and I lost control of my emotions and started to cry. David had never heard me cry before. None of my children had ever seen or heard me cry. At this point in the conversation, I lost all semblance of composure. The only words that I could force through my lips were "David! I am very sick!" Then I was crying uncontrollably, and I handed the telephone to Wendy. She told David everything. They talked for a long time.

I felt as if my life were crumbling. Everything was closing in on me, and I had no answers and no control over what was happening to me and my family. Wendy sat down on the couch beside me. She dried my eyes and cheeks with a paper napkin, put her arms around me, and kissed me. She told me about her conversation with David. He was going to immediately call his brother and sisters, tell them what had happened to me, and then he would catch the next flight out to Wilmington.

I felt relieved. I had been worried about how I was going to tell my family. I had been carrying the weight of this emotional burden, and it had been constantly on my mind. Now that problem was gone. I sat there with Wendy. She was holding me in her arms, and I could feel her love flowing through my body.

The telephone rang most of that evening, as each of my children called. I was unable to speak to them, so Wendy explained about what the tests had indicated and what the doctor had said. They told Wendy that they were making travel arrangements and would be arriving that weekend, except Pam, who lived in Charleston, South Carolina, with her husband and one-and-a-half-year-old daughter, Lauren. Pam was seven months' pregnant and was unable to travel.

The fact that I would be seeing them very soon was wonderful, but I knew that this was just the beginning of my burden on each of them. Their lives would be changed because of my illness, and that bothered me.

I had been extremely independent and in control of my life. Now, all of a sudden, everything had changed. Instead of my being the one that each of my children could come to if they had a problem or needed help, now I had become someone that they would worry about. Certainly their concern would affect their lives in a negative way. The thought of such a role reversal was very upsetting to me.

My mind flashed back to the years past, starting with one of my children and then another. I recalled the many experiences that each of them had been through as part of growing up. Whenever and wherever I could help them, I had always tried to do my best, and, since our marriage, Wendy had always been very supportive of my efforts to give assistance.

I jumped, as Wendy put her head on my shoulder. I was sitting on the couch and had been so engrossed in my memories that I had forgotten where I was and what was happening to me.

Wendy said, "You have been through a lot this evening, and I am glad that the children know about the illness. Even under such circumstances, it will be wonderful to have the whole family together again. You look tired. Why don't you get some rest." She walked with me to the bedroom and helped me get undressed, and then she got my sleeping pills and a cup of water with a straw. Soon, she tucked me into bed and gave me a good night kiss.

Friday morning came, and Amanda was at school. She was excited about the news that her brothers and sister would be arriving that weekend. She said she couldn't wait to get through with her school day and return home. Of course, Amanda did not understand why they were coming. Wendy and I had decided not to alarm her about my illness, especially when we didn't have any answers to the many questions that she would ask.

My physical condition worsened; my symptoms seemed to be moving along quite rapidly. I was losing weight. I could eat only soft foods that required very little chewing, often mixing whatever I ate with some kind of gravy. There were fasciculations in my tongue, my throat, my arms, and my legs. Swallowing had become very difficult, and I was having constant problems with my saliva. There was very little energy left in my body, and I would tire easily from the simplest of tasks, such as trying to brush my hair or getting dressed.

Needless to say, I had mixed emotions about the upcoming family get-together. Certainly, I was excited about seeing my children, but things would be different this time. Instead of it being a joyous, happy occasion filled with laughter and exciting conversation about what was going on in everyone's life, it was bound to be different. But I couldn't imagine what it would be like. How would my older children respond to me? How would I respond?

The rest of the day, I tried to gain my composure and decide exactly how I would manage the situation. I went over and over various scenarios in my mind, trying to decide what I could say or how I could explain what was happening to me. I began to realize that my emotional state would make it impossible for me to be in control of the situation. I was frightened, really frightened. This was a feeling that was foreign to me, real fear. I had always been a take-charge person. I would just jump right into a situation, identify the problem, and take action. Then I would develop a solution and implement it. But how could I apply my strategy to what was happening to my health, my body, my life? I was dying, and it would happen in slow motion, dragged out over months of deterioration, despair, and suffering—not only suffering for me but suffering for the entire family. How can I be the father, the husband, the man of the family under these circumstances? I saw myself as a helpless victim who would slowly decay like a fallen tree.

Wendy walked into the family room where I was sitting. She gently reached out for my hand and helped me get up from the couch. We went out on the patio and she asked how I was feeling. Tears started to flow down my cheeks because I hurt very badly inside. Completely losing my composure allowed me to open up, and I told her about my thoughts and concerns. Suddenly I realized that my illness was not only affecting my body but also beginning to invade my mind. I felt as if I were drowning.

Wendy took me in her arms and held me, while she talked about love and caring and about how the older children were young adults now and in control of their own lives. "You can let go of the feeling that you have to be responsible for every aspect of their lives or even your own right now," she reassured me. A feeling of peace came over me, and I began to calm down as she looked into my eyes and said, "I will take care of everything, dear." Then she led me back into the house and to our bedroom, where I could rest until Amanda returned from school.

When my eyes opened, Wendy was sitting on the bed gently touching my arm. Amanda had long been home from school, Debbie had arrived from Salisbury, and David, Jr., had arrived from the local airport after renting a car. Mike would be flying in on Sunday. Everything was arranged, and now it was time for me to get myself together. Wendy helped me brush my hair and put on my bathrobe. She smiled at me, giving me a hug and a loving kiss on the cheek. "Everything will be all right," she said. My wonderful Wendy took my arm, and we started down the hallway. I was nervous and filled with apprehension. Even though I had been resting in bed for several hours, my legs were weak. In fact, I was having trouble mustering energy throughout my entire body. Then I felt Wendy's hand under my arm, and I felt confident that I could rise to the occasion.

Debbie, David, and Amanda were all sitting at the kitchen table. Some of Amanda's drawings from school were the subject of the conversation. They were very colorful drawings filled with splashes of bright red, dark green, deep blue, and a glowing yellow. As Wendy and I walked into the kitchen, Debbie and David quickly turned to greet us, and Amanda asked me to sit down at the table and look at her artwork. Wendy joined the group as Amanda started to tell me all about the pictures she had drawn and what she had eaten for lunch at school and about the new boy in her class. It was a pleasant conversation and helped everyone to relax and feel comfortable.

We all used Amanda as the center of our focus. Our conversation was light and general for a while, and then Amanda grew restless and wanted to play outside. She placed her school papers on the kitchen counter and out the door she went, singing a song she had learned at school.

Each of the family members took turns asking questions. I brought Debbie and David up to date regarding my medical prognosis, and even though my speech was weak and somewhat slurred, we communicated well. My energy level was good for the first time in several weeks. Seeing Debbie and David had energized my mind and body, and the apprehension that had taunted my mind was gone. I was excited about having the family together. Wendy took Amanda along with her to the grocery store so that Amanda wouldn't have to be involved in such a serious matter until we really knew what was happening.

Amanda was a happy child and so curious about everything new that she saw or heard discussed. I was worried about how all this would affect her. She is my little miracle child, and I love her deeply. Before marrying, Wendy and I had discussed, in great detail, the fact that neither one of us wanted to have children. Wendy was involved in a very successful career that had vaulted her into a high-profile executive position with an international corporation, and she really didn't have any motherly instinct. I had started my first marriage at age nineteen and had already been through the responsibilities of raising children, or at least to the best of my ability at the time. My first wife and I were both too young and inexperienced in life to do a really good job as parents. I was thankful that our children had survived and achieved success through our love and their fortitude. So, needless to say, I was not interested in starting over as a new parent at this point in my life. But out of the blue one morning, after Wendy and I had been married about three years, she told me during breakfast that she wanted to be a mother. To say that I was surprised would certainly be an understatement. But I could see by the look on her face and sense by the tone of her voice that becoming a mother was something that had become very meaningful for her. Thus, our little miracle, Amanda, came into our lives.

During dinner, I used my neck collar to help support my head. I had several cans of Ensure, which the doctor had prescribed for me. I did very little talking and found myself growing weaker. Keeping my throat clear was becoming a problem. Suddenly, I became aware of the stress that I was experiencing; my mind was racing with many different thoughts. What was going to happen to me? How were Wendy and Amanda going to deal with my illness? Would I be dead soon? What could I do to make all this go away? The tears were beginning to well up in my eyes. Using the strongest voice I could muster, I excused myself and Wendy walked with me back to our bedroom. She helped me get my robe off. By this time, I was very weak and took my medicine and went to bed. Wendy stayed with me for a while. Then she said, "I want to get Amanda ready for bed and then spend some time with Debbie and David, but I promise to look in on you later to see how you are doing." She kissed me, smiled, and left the room.

Saturday was not a very good day for me. I spent most of the day lying down. It was becoming harder for me to keep my throat clear. My speech was very labored, and even drinking the Ensure through a straw was a difficult task. My mind was cluttered with so many thoughts, all jumbled up. There were thoughts about my older children when they were young, and I could see scenes from the past flashing through my mind.

Sunday was not any better, and when my oldest son, Mike, arrived, I talked with him for a while, but my throat problem worsened and caused me to head back to bed. Fear started to well up within me again. I felt as if I were choking, and Wendy tried to adjust the angle of my head, but nothing seemed to work. She could see that I was having great difficulty and decided to phone the doctor. She explained what had taken place over the last few days, regarding my throat, and that I seemed to be choking at times. The doctor told Wendy to bring me to the hospital emergency room and that he would meet us there. Wendy gave me a quick shower in the special chair that fit into the bathtub, making the shower less demanding for me. Clothed in clean pajamas, a bathrobe, and slippers, I was helped to the car and driven to the hospital to meet my neurologist.

After a quick examination, the doctor made arrangements for me to be admitted as an inpatient. I underwent a series of X-rays and laboratory tests, including blood work. My energy was depleted. I was originally placed in a wheelchair, but I was unable to hold my head up, even with the neck collar that I used, and my upper body was bent over the right arm support of the wheelchair. The nurses decided to transfer me to a rolling stretcher for the duration of time required to complete all the tests that the doctor had ordered. The area of the hospital that I was located in was very cold, and even though the nurses had placed two blankets over me, I could feel the coldness piercing my body. It seemed to pass into my bones, and then my body started shivering to the point that one of the nurses, who was wearing a thick green sweater, brought me another blanket.

I was taken to my hospital room. A nurse came in with the doctor and set up a suction device that I could use to help keep my mouth clear. Much was happening to my body, but I guess that was to be expected. I couldn't seem to get over being scared. Not having much experience with the emotion of fear left me at a great disadvantage because I had no basic coping skills to apply to the problem. Maybe that was a starting point for me to work with. After all, my illness didn't produce the fear; my thoughts were the culprit. Knowing that my family had come to spend time with me and that I had ended up in the hospital evoked another emotion that I was more familiar with: frustration. I was frustrated with myself for not being emotionally stronger, but it was all very depressing. What could I do? Was there anything that the doctors could do?

Everything had been going so well in my life. Wendy and I had worked hard to get to the point where we could move to Florida and begin our new family adventure. We had many dreams and plans for the future. What was happening to me was not fair! And it wasn't fair to Wendy and Amanda. All our dreams were disappearing, as our lives were ravaged by this disease. How could it be?

Amyotrophic lateral sclerosis (ALS), more commonly known in this country as Lou Gehrig's disease, was discovered over 120 years ago, and tens of thousands of people have died from it. Yet medical science doesn't even know what causes it. There is no medication or treatment to even slow the progression, and doctors say there is absolutely nothing that can be done. How can this be, when science can split an atom, fertilize a human egg that grows into a healthy living baby, and send men to the moon and bring them safely back to earth? How can this disease continue to ravage humankind for so many years, with scientists not even knowing where to begin!

7

Three days had gone by, and the medication the doctor had prescribed to reduce the flow of saliva was working. I was still hooked up to the intravenous feeding tube, because I was unable to chew and swallow solid food. I was on a liquid diet and was able to take thick fluids by mouth, such as creamed soups, mashed potatoes covered with gravy, applesauce, and pudding. Anything that was fluid in consistency but had no solids mixed in could be swallowed.

The main concern was that I might aspirate the food, meaning that some might get into my windpipe and cause me to choke or might end up in my lungs.

The doctors had found, during the many tests and examinations that had been performed on me, that my palate was completely paralyzed and nonfunctional. A therapist had been working with me so that I could learn how to swallow safely, thus reducing the chance that I might aspirate when taking in my liquid food. We had started with a mixture of liquid and small pieces of solid food but quickly found that I just couldn't handle anything other than thick liquids.

The therapist taught me to use a chewing motion, even though I was taking in only liquids. The chewing motion made it easier for me to swallow and also helped to produce natural digestive juices in my mouth as well as my stomach.

I was distracted from my thoughts by the sound of the doctor entering my room. He wrote something on a medical chart and then walked over to my bed, put his hand on my arm, and smiled. I was thinking how fortunate I was to have a doctor who actually took time to be warm and caring. So many of the other doctors and nurses I have encountered have been impersonal, cold, even uncaring. Yes, I was fortunate to be under the medical care of a doctor who took time to talk, to listen, and to care enough to offer a warm smile and a reassuring touch.

We talked for a while. He asked how I was feeling and wanted to know if the medication was helping and whether or not I was experiencing any new problems. I replied to each of his inquiries, relating my concerns about what would happen to me next and where I would go from this point in time. I knew that he really didn't have the answer to what I was asking. I guess I was just thinking out loud.

The expression on my doctor's face changed from a warm, pleasant smile to a more serious but still friendly appearance. He glanced at my medical chart, which he was holding in his left hand and said, "Because of your condition, I believe it would be prudent for us to explore some of the possibilities that you might face in the foreseeable future." He went on to say he had made arrangements for two other doctors to visit me later in the day. One would discuss my breathing and swallowing problems, and the other doctor would present some potential solutions to some of the challenges that I would face in the future.

Our discussion was interrupted by a nurse who was there to check what she referred to as my vital signs. My doctor moved back a few steps from the bed so that the nurse could hook me up to the blood pressure equipment, place a thermometer in my mouth, and check my pulse.

As I was lying there waiting for the thermometer to beep, my eyes scanned the nurse's face. It was expressionless, almost mechanical in appearance, in spite of her pretty blue eyes and attractive hair style. She was around twenty-two or twenty-three years old and was a well-groomed woman, yet the mechanical appearance of her face and the staccato movements of her hands and arms, along with her general body language, gave the appearance of a robot. It was as if she were just another piece of medical equipment in the room.

The sound of the beep from the thermometer startled me, I had been so engrossed in my observation of the nurse. She quickly finished her notations on my medical chart, which the doctor had laid on the bedside table. She turned, having never made eye contact with me, and said, "Thank you, doctor," and then left the room.

Just as suddenly as the nurse had passed through the doorway, a middle-aged lady came into my room carrying a tray. She removed the cover and then left the room. It was lunch time, and my tray contained the usual—two large cups of flavored broth, a flexible straw, and a dish of very soft pudding. My doctor rose to his feet, walked over to my bed, patted my arm, and smiled. "Remember, you will be seeing the two doctors whom we spoke about earlier. They should be in to visit with you around 2:30 to 3:00 this afternoon," he said, as he waved and turned to leave the room.

With the door closed, the room was very quiet. My neck felt weak, and I had very little energy left, so I decided to just lie there and try to think things through. My mind began to wander, and questions about my illness swirled around in my head. I knew I didn't have any answers to these medical questions and neither did the doctors. This process was just making me feel worse, so I decided I would concentrate on something pleasant. Scenes of Florida gently filled my mind—beautiful, warm weather, the bright colors of flowers, the deep green of tropical foliage, and the blue water of the ocean rushing toward the soft white sand on the beach. Wendy, Amanda, and I were there on the beach having fun, and we were all happy.

A knock on the door startled me. As I slowly turned my head, the door opened, and a rather short man wearing a white coat entered my room. He introduced himself. This was one of the doctors my neurologist had said would visit me. He was followed by a nurse pushing a rolling cart that contained a number of items, all packaged in plastic.

This was a nurse that I hadn't encountered before. She had a very pleasant smile and looked me directly in the eye. Her demeanor was reassuring as well as comforting. The doctor approached my bed and said, "I am here at the request of your neurologist to discuss options regarding your eating problem and to demonstrate some equipment that can alleviate some of the difficulties that you are experiencing."

He discussed the problems that could develop and how they would affect my normal intake of food and medicine. "We must protect you from any possibility of aspirating food or liquid," he continued, "and the feeding devices or tubes that I have here can safely solve any such problem."

As he spoke, the nurse opened the plastic packs and

handed each item to the doctor. I was in a daze, and the doctor's voice was audible to me, but I really didn't hear what he was saying. Nor did I focus on the items that he was displaying. The doctor's voice seemed to be like a deep, monotone, humming sound. I could hear the words coming from his mouth, but what he was saying sounded like a very slow-speed recording. Suddenly the tone of his voice changed, as he held in his right hand one of the devices. "This is your very best option," he said. "We make an incision through your side, adjacent to your stomach, and then into the stomach itself. This device is inserted through the incision and into your stomach. All your nourishment, medication—whatever—is passed through this peg-tube directly into your stomach so that you don't have to worry about chewing and swallowing. This procedure is known as a gastrostomy. After a short period of time, the peg is adjusted and has a cap that fits snugly. No one will even know it's there, even if you are wearing a bathing suit!"

I looked at his face. He seemed very pleased with the peg device he held up for me to look at. "Do you have any questions about what I have explained to you, or is there anything you would like me to go over again?" he asked. My mind was filled with questions. So I started asking, "Is this permanent?" The doctor's facial expression changed as he answered, "Under the progressive degeneration regarding your illness, I would think you would want to continue to use the peg, but it can be removed and the incision can be closed with stitches, leaving very little external scarring."

"Will I still be able to take food or liquid by mouth?" I asked. "Yes," he replied. "But that could create problems regarding aspiration of foreign substances into your lungs, and also there is always the possibility of pneumonia. That is a very serious complication for a patient with ALS."

My head was spinning. Things were moving too fast. My voice grew weaker as I asked, "Doctor, when would I have to have this done? I mean, not now! Maybe sometime in the future?" His reply didn't answer my question. "It would be best if you talked to your neurologist about the timing, but in my opinion there is no reason to take any unnecessary chances," he said.

Our conversation was interrupted by the second doctor. He entered the room with an older man who was pushing a large rolling cart, much larger in size than the cart with the feeding apparatus. "Am I too early?" the other doctor asked. The short doctor turned to me and said, "If you have additional questions after you have spoken with your neurologist, here is my card. Call me anytime." He turned to the nurse, who had placed all the items back into their plastic packs and told her it was time to go. He looked back at me and said, "Please, don't hesitate to call if I can be of any further assistance." He then stepped toward the doorway and spoke briefly with the other doctor. The nurse turned and left the room with the small rolling cart.

The older man had moved his cart to the foot of my bed. There were a number of strange-looking apparatuses on the top shelf, as well as items on a lower shelf. I guessed this older man was a nurse or maybe a technician of some kind. He didn't speak but just stood there with his hands resting on the cart.

The second doctor walked over to my bed and introduced himself but made no attempt to shake my hand or make any physical gesture. He said, "Your neurologist asked me to visit with you, and I brought along some equipment that is used in assisting patients with their breathing. I have some very basic breathing equipment that assists normal breathing patterns, as well as more sophisticated units that breathe for you as your disease progresses.

"I have read your chart and the results of the breathing test that you have been taking twice a day. It seems, at this point in time, that your breathing capacity is labored but adequate. But as time passes, ALS patients require more assistance and eventually need to be placed on a ventilator. In fact, I have a number of ALS patients that are living at home and using ventilators very successfully."

I stared at the doctor's face. He was wearing eyeglasses that rested halfway down his nose, and he was peering at me over them. His expression was very similar to that of the nurse who took my blood pressure and temperature, almost expressionless and mechanical in appearance.

My body was approaching exhaustion, and my mind was jumping from thoughts of my family to my high school days to flashes of Wendy and me when we were dating.

The doctor's voice caught my attention as he said, "Mr. Atkinson, are you ready to get started? Are there any questions that you would like to ask me?" I knew that I must get some rest from the thoughts of feeding tubes and breathing equipment and everything else that I was being bombarded with.

My thoughts turned to visiting hours. My family would be arriving that evening to visit with me, and I needed to rest, so I could sit up in bed and talk with them and look strong and alert.

Debbie had to get back to her new job and to her son Neal and daughter Nicole. Mike, who was general manager of a large resort property that included four restaurants, would be flying back early tomorrow. David was flying out tomorrow afternoon to return to his law practice. They had come to spend time with me and to help in any way that they could. Instead of us all being together during this difficult time, our time together had been reduced to a few hours in a hospital room. Once again, the doctor's voice penetrated my consciousness. He said, "Mr. Atkinson, we really must get started!" There was no way that I could deal with any more pressure, and I wasn't sure that I wanted any more information about breathing equipment. I responded to the doctor, "Please, I am very tired. I can't absorb what you are telling me. Please, take all this stuff away and leave me alone!" The doctor started to speak, but I interrupted him. "Please, just go away, go away. I can't take any more of this!" I exclaimed. Then I rolled over on my side, away from the doctor, and buried my head in the pillow.

First there was the sound of muffled voices, then the squeaking sound of the wheels on the rolling cart. They were leaving my room and taking their equipment with them. A sense of relief fell over me. Now, maybe I could get some rest and prepare myself to see my family during visiting hours.

After sleeping for a while, I felt a little better. Everyone was there and they chatted away while I relaxed and just listened. Time passed quickly, and I knew I wouldn't be seeing my older children for a while because they had to return to their homes. They couldn't be expected to put their lives on hold and sit around with me day in and day out.

Three more days passed, and the doctor discharged me from the hospital. Then I was back home with Wendy and Amanda. My three older children had said goodbye and left town for their respective homes. I felt guilty, knowing they had each set aside their individual responsibilities and rushed here to be with me. It was disappointing that we had spent very little time together because I was in the hospital.

My doctor had not mentioned anything about the episode regarding the breathing apparatus demonstration, and neither had I. He had decided to have me return home, because there wasn't anything more that could be done for me at the hospital.

Wendy was taking care of me, and I was living on Ensure and strained baby food. I used the neck collar during the day to support my head for those periods of time when I would sit in the family room or living room and at the table during mealtime.

My doctor had scheduled a series of tests and Wendy drove me to the outpatient department at the hospital and various other doctors' offices, as well as my neurologist's office. Some of the tests were to determine the strength of my throat muscles in order to establish whether or not they were still strong enough to keep my air passage open. Others were to monitor my breathing, and the purpose of additional testing has faded from my memory.

The neurosurgeon at Chapel Hill was scheduled to perform my nerve and muscle biopsies the next day at 11:30 a.m. Wendy would be driving me the two-and-a-half hours to Chapel Hill, where I would be an outpatient at the University of North Carolina Hospital. I was thankful that there was no need for me to spend the night in the hospital. To me this meant that the biopsy procedures must be simple and not considered dangerous.

We owned an Oldsmobile station wagon with a back seat that could be folded down. Using a number of blankets and a pillow, Wendy made a comfortable bed for me to use during the trip to and from Chapel Hill. I knew that it would be a long and tiring day for me, but I was looking forward to meeting this doctor who had extensive experience with the ALS disease. Maybe the biopsies would indicate that I didn't have ALS! Maybe he would find that I had a less serious illness that could be successfully treated.

We arrived an hour early for my appointment. I was

well rested, because I had taken an extra sleeping pill the night before and was able to rest comfortably during the trip. I wanted to make a good impression on this new doctor. I had dressed in very casual clothes, and even though I had to wear the neck collar to support my head, I wanted to appear as if I were doing just fine. If he didn't see me as an ALS patient, maybe he would be more likely to look for another illness.

This new neurologist turned out to be a very congenial person. He had a pleasant smile, and his attitude was on the light side. I felt very comfortable and relaxed during his brief examination. In fact, I had only to remove my shoes and socks and lie on my stomach on a small table. The doctor explained exactly what he was going to do and how he was going to do it. There was one nurse who was assisting him with the biopsies. First, he gave me several injections of a local anesthetic in my right lower ankle. The nurse cleaned the area and placed some material over it to create a sterile field. Because of my position on the table, I was unable to observe the procedure, but the doctor talked me through everything he did. "I will make a very small incision, and then I will remove some nerve tissue and some muscle tissue. You will have a very small area on the side of your foot where there will be no sensation after the nerve tissue is removed, but this procedure will not affect your physical ability in any manner whatsoever," he explained.

His next words came as a surprise to me when he said, "I have both the samples of tissue that I need. Now we will close the incision with several sutures and cover it with a protective bandage."

The procedure was over quickly, and there was no pain. Wendy had been sitting on a tall stool just a few feet away and had been able to observe everything. She walked over and held my hand while the nurse applied the bandage. I was thinking how much I liked the way this doctor had dealt with me and how well I related to him.

I motioned for Wendy to lean toward me, and then I whispered, "The doctor has a nice English accent just like yours, dear." Wendy responded emphatically, "That's not an English accent. He's from Scotland!" Just then, the doctor walked over and handed Wendy an instruction sheet regarding the care of my ankle. He said, "Your neurologist in Wilmington will remove the sutures and will examine the incision for proper healing." Wendy spoke up, "What part of Scotland do you call home?" Wendy and the doctor talked while the nurse helped me sit up and put on my socks and shoes.

We arrived home late that afternoon. I'm not sure whether I slept during the drive home or not, but by the time we got into the house, I was feeling beat. Wendy helped me to our bedroom, took my shoes off, and helped me remove my neck collar. Then I lay down on the bed to rest, and Wendy gave me a kiss and a warm smile. I reached out and took her hand, saying, "Thank you for loving me and caring so much about me. After all that driving, I know you must be very tired. Why don't you lie down and rest for a while?" She sat down on the edge of the bed and caressed my arm, looking directly into my eyes. She said, "I will always be here for you, David." She gently let go of my hand, stood up, and headed down the hallway toward the kitchen.

As I lay there in bed, my mind started to race with many thoughts about different events. Some of my thoughts made sense, and others seemed to come from out of the blue.

It had now been twenty-seven days since I left the manufacturing plant and Wendy left the furniture store. By this point in time, our plans called for us to be settled into our new lifestyle in Florida. Amanda would have been attending her new school, and Wendy and I would have started a new business venture or at least would be preparing to launch our new business.

It was hard to believe that twenty-seven days had slipped away from us. But even more difficult to comprehend was the amount of money that had slipped away! All this time, there had been no family income, but there had been our regular daily living expenses plus numerous unexpected bills to pay. My prescription cost had gone up dramatically. Then there was the twenty percent that we had to pay for all my medical expenses that were not covered by my hospitalization insurance.

Hospitalization insurance! Suddenly the thought hit me like a bolt of lighting. My insurance coverage would end thirty days from the last day that my name appeared on the payroll records. I was aware of the thirty-day clause, regarding my hospitalization insurance, but that had not been a major concern, because I thought for sure that I would have a new business set up before the thirty-day period ran out. Also, I knew that we could get nonbusiness coverage for the family until insurance would be available through the business, if that were necessary. No one in the family had had any medical problems, so we counted on qualifying for a family policy at a reasonable rate.

My heart was pounding, and I was sweating profusely. How could I have forgotten about the thirty-day grace period? Twenty-seven days had vanished, and that meant I had only three days left of insurance coverage! Not only would I have no insurance coverage, but neither would Wendy or Amanda. My first thought was to telephone one of my former partners. Then I realized that they wouldn't have any answers. They would have to get in touch with the company's insurance agent. So I telephoned the insurance agent directly and explained my situation. He said, "I'll have to make a few calls and find out what can be done." He would telephone me back just as soon as he had some answers.

Wendy was in the laundry room using the washer and dryer. My first thought was to tell her about the insurance situation, but then I realized there was nothing she could do about it, other than to have one more serious problem to worry about. She was under a lot of stress, so I decided to get this problem solved on my own. I waited for the insurance agent to call me back.

It seemed as though two or three hours had passed, but actually it had been only about forty-five minutes since I talked with the agent. I waited another half hour, then telephoned him again. His voice was rather weak. "I've made several calls—one to the area supervisor and another to the home office. I'm waiting for them to call me back, and just as soon as they do, I'll call you," he said. The rest of the afternoon was spent waiting for the telephone to ring. There were two calls that afternoon, but not the one that I hoped for.

At 9:00 a.m. the next morning, on day twenty-nine I telephoned the insurance office. The agent was not there but was expected around 9:30. The woman who answered the telephone assured me that she would have him call me just as soon as he arrived.

Wendy was in the garage going through some boxes, when the telephone rang at 9:55. It was the insurance agent. He went into great detail about what he had learned. Every possibility had been explored, and there was nothing that could be done to extend my insurance coverage. The insurance company was already aware of my illness, because they had been paying eighty percent of my claims for the last several weeks. So not only would they not extend my coverage period, but they would not write any new coverage. They would consider writing coverage for Wendy and Amanda, but a new application form must be completed and forwarded to the underwriter.

The agent explained that there was a federal regulation, referred to as the COBRA law, which allowed an individual in my situation to automatically receive extended coverage from his insurance carrier for eighteen months, and then the possibility of some additional time beyond the eighteen months. Of course, the premium would be much higher than the group rate, but at least there would be coverage. However, the insurance company was contesting my eligibility to qualify for COBRA coverage. There was a rule stating that for an employee to qualify for COBRA, the company he worked for must have more than twenty-one employees. "Well, what's the problem?" I asked. "Our company has more than forty employees!"

As it turned out, there were two companies. When we first opened our business, we formed the original company, which included the partners, or stockholders, because we were incorporated. As the business expanded, a second company was formed to include an acquisition. But we continued to pay the upper management people along with several of the office personnel from the original company. Thus, the insurance company was able to have me declared ineligible for COBRA coverage.

After exhausting every legal avenue that was open to me, I finally had to accept that, technically, the insurance company was correct. I informed Wendy of our plight. We did secure hospitalization coverage for Wendy and Amanda with Blue Cross, but the premium was very expensive.

My medical bills continued, and without insurance we had to pay, personally, for every prescription, every doctor's bill, and every lab test and procedure. Our financial reserve was disappearing rapidly, and according to the expected progression of the disease, the big expenses were yet to come.

During this very bleak time in our lives, there was one very meaningful and caring gesture that will remain fresh in my mind for the rest of my days on this earth. When my local neurologist in Wilmington found out about what had happened with my hospitalization insurance, he expressed his disgust for the insurance company's actions, but more important were his actions. He instructed his office staff not to bill me for any additional services and also told them not to accept any payment from us for bills that were previously due. He continued to see me on a regular basis and refused to accept any further payment.

Days turned into weeks, and before we knew what had hit us, we were financially broke. Everything that we had worked so hard for was gone. For a short period of time, we paid our bills using credit cards, thinking somehow something good would happen, but reality finally set in. We stopped using our credit cards, even though there were still a couple of thousand dollars available on our credit line. We knew that we could not continue to live this way any longer. It was decision time.

8

My disease progressed rapidly. The muscle and nerve biopsies showed nerve and muscle degeneration indicative of ALS. There came a day when my neurologist told me that in his opinion I had about six months or maybe less before I would require a feeding tube and, most likely, a ventilator. He suggested that I prepare myself and my family for what was ahead.

I had a living will stating that my life was not to be extended by artificial means. This meant that I was facing about six months more to live.

My older children had been in touch with us on a regular basis and had all offered to help us financially, but after seeing what had happened to our financial reserves in a relatively short period of time, I said no.

Our financial requirements had turned into a bottomless pit, and my medical prognosis would mean much larger medical expenses in the months to come. I was not willing to let this disease financially drain my entire family.

We now knew that we would never move to Florida. There had been much discussion among all the family members as to what we should do during the next six months.

The first problem that had to be addressed immediately was our financial situation. For the first time in our lives, we were past due on our bills. We received letters and phone calls dunning us for payments. We wrote to each company that we owed and explained about my medical condition and what had happened to us financially. But rather than persuading our creditors to hold off until arrangements could be made for payment in the future, our letter caused a feeding frenzy, and all the creditors tried to get their money immediately.

We contacted a local attorney to see what could be done to stop what had turned into daily harassment by many of our creditors. After meeting with the attorney, we discovered that, in addition to our personal debt, the notes Wendy and I had signed when we were shareholders in the manufacturing business were also listed against us. We had thought when we sold our interest in the business that because we no longer had any ownership, our business liabilities would cease. We had sent a letter to each business creditor, notifying them that we were selling our interest in the business and would no longer be responsible for any of the business debts. Not one of those business creditors ever responded to our letter to say that our obligation still existed.

There seemed only one way to legally stop the letters, phone calls, and harassment: bankruptcy. When I first heard about the recommendation of bankruptcy, I was stunned. On top of everything else that was happening, I was being reduced to the level of a deadbeat. I had always believed that there was no legitimate reason for anyone filing for bankruptcy. It was just a technical loophole for people and companies to beat the system.

After many conversations with my son, I finally understood and halfheartedly accepted that I would have to file for bankruptcy. But under the law, I could not file just in my name; Wendy would have to be included. So I would have to live with this stigma for about six months, while Wendy would have to live with it for the rest of her life. How unfair life had become! We had hit bottom, or at least that's what I thought at that point in time.

There was a general consensus among the family—and I agreed—that Wendy, Amanda, and I should move to Salisbury, North Carolina, where Debbie lived. The reasoning was that we were going to be facing a horrendous six months to come, and with Debbie's professional training as a psychotherapist and her experience in dealing with families experiencing catastrophes in their lives, she would be best equipped to help Wendy and Amanda through this very difficult period of time. Also, Debbie would be of great assistance to me, because she was already well versed and knowledgeable regarding exactly the kind of care that I would need as my disease progressed.

So it was decided that we would move to Salisbury. By this point in time, I was very weak and physically unable to do any lifting. It seemed that I was best at just taking up space and getting in the way. It was extremely difficult for me to watch Wendy have to meet all our daily needs, as well as prepare for our move north, rather than south, as originally planned.

Events moved along rapidly. Several of our friends, including my brother-in-law, Bill, helped load what personal items we still owned into a rental truck. Bill and I had been friends for more than twenty years. We had been very close for a number of years, and I still thought of him as a brother. He was a true gentleman and probably the most talented individual that I had ever known, and I certainly would miss him. Bill was the husband of my first wife's sister.

My older children helped financially, so we had enough money for a deposit and the rent on a very small two-bedroom apartment in Salisbury. But, once again, everything seemed to be going downhill for us. When we arrived at the apartment complex, Wendy went into the rental office. Soon, she came out of the office with a lease for me to sign just below her signature. I noticed that she looked very tense, so I asked, "What's the matter?" She pointed at a clause on the page of the lease that I had just signed. As I read it, my mind started to swirl. In bold type were printed these words: "Before this lease is accepted we are required to secure a credit report for all applicants named in this lease." Wendy spoke up, "They run the credit check on a machine in the office. The lady said it would take about fifteen minutes, and if there were no problems, we could start to move in."

We had three of our friends who had driven the truck to Salisbury waiting to unload everything and help Wendy get the apartment set up. Then they would be returning the truck to the nearest dealer. One of them had driven his car, so they would all have a way to get back to Wilmington. If we were turned down for the apartment because of our credit report, it would truly be a disaster. We would have a truck that we were paying for by the day, filled with our personal belongings, and three friends who had to leave very soon and return to Wilmington.

Wendy and I talked for a couple of minutes. We decided that we had nothing to lose at this point, except the twenty-five-dollar nonrefundable fee for securing the credit report.

As I lay in the car, Wendy explained to the rental agent that I was ill and it would be easier for me not to go into the office to complete any paperwork. It seemed as if two hours or more passed by. Finally, I could see Wendy emerging from the rental office. She walked over, smiled, and gave me a loving hug. Everything was approved. The credit report had come back indicating that we were credit worthy! I found out sometime later that because we had filed for bankruptcy, none of the creditors were permitted to list our debts with the credit bureau, and the bankruptcy itself had not been officially recorded. Seven days later and we would not have qualified.

We had never lived in an apartment before and discovered quickly that even though we didn't have a lot of personal belongings left, there still wasn't room for what we did have. We were able to find an inexpensive storage space nearby that solved the problem. We had one bathroom, and if any two of us went down the hallway at the same time, we had to turn sideways to pass. This was our new home, but at least we had some place safe and convenient to live.

Amanda was excited, because the complex had a nice swimming pool for the tenants and she was looking forward to meeting the other children who lived there. As it turned out, there were approximately 130 apartments and only one other child close to Amanda's age—a boy. But they became friends, and swimming kept Amanda occupied. Fortunately, she would be starting school in three weeks and would meet new friends and teachers.

After a week of settling in, Wendy and I set up a schedule. She helped me bathe and get dressed. Then I would have puréed food and my Ensure for breakfast. Wendy would have something already prepared for my lunch, and then she would leave. She hoped to find a part-time job that would fit in with my needs at home. I would be there each day when Amanda was dropped off by the school bus, just a couple of units from ours.

Amanda's use of the pool was short-lived. The temperatures dropped, as fall and then winter set upon us. I found that I was affected much more severely by the colder temperatures than before my illness. I seemed to stay cold most of the time, and my travels outside of the apartment were minimal.

Wendy had difficulty finding any type of job. There weren't many jobs available, but the biggest drawbacks were Wendy's years of experience and her previous salary level. No one wanted to hire her for the jobs that were available because they knew she was overqualified and assumed that she would leave just as soon as she found a more appropriate job.

We could not continue to draw upon the older children's resources. They all had their own responsibilities to manage, and we had to get through this on our own. I was eligible for a Social Security disability payment because my illness was terminal and the payment had already been approved while we were living in Wilmington. But Social Security's rules required a six-month waiting period before the payments would start, and it was not retroactive. Also, there was a twenty-four-month waiting period before I would qualify under Medicare disability for any type of medical coverage. So it looked as if all that money I had paid to Social Security over the years would be given to someone else.

Both Wendy and I were ineligible for unemployment payments, even though thousands of dollars had been paid for unemployment insurance over the years. In my case, my illness disqualified me, because I had to be seeking new employment in order to qualify. In Wendy's case, the fact that she had left her job voluntarily disqualified her.

After weeks of fighting the thought of filing for Medicaid, food stamps, and the other welfare programs that we were eligible for, the decision was made. We had no other choice. We had to pay our rent and buy food, and address all the other normal family expenses, as well as my medical expenses. It was hard to believe what had happened to us in a relatively short period of time.

We had worked hard and were able to live a very comfortable lifestyle. It was mind-boggling: we went from para-sailing in Acapulco, Mexico, to welfare in Salisbury!

I had seen several doctors since moving to Salisbury and would soon have to locate a dentist. It was difficult finding doctors or dentists who would accept Medicaid patients. I was assigned a Social Services caseworker who was very nice but not very effective. It was difficult getting a definitive answer to what seemed to be a very simple question. Later on in the process, I was fortunate to be assigned a very professional and capable caseworker, and I will be forever thankful to Mrs. R. for her understanding and compassion and for really caring about me and my family.

There was not a neurologist in Salisbury—amazing but true. I contacted my friend and former neurologist in Wilmington and asked if he knew of anyone close to Salisbury that he could recommend. He said he would make some contacts and let me know.

Finally, something good happened. As it turned out, the specialist who had come so highly recommended and who had done my biopsies agreed to see me as a clinic patient in Chapel Hill. Both Wendy and I had liked him very much, and I was excited about having Dr. H. as my neurologist.

Even though Chapel Hill was about one and three-quarters of an hour from Salisbury, the drive there was on interstate highway. Medicaid would pay for my medical expenses, medication, and something toward transportation, because I was being seen in a clinic at a teaching hospital.

Wendy and I used the same arrangement that we had before, regarding a place for me to lie down in the back of the station wagon. When we arrived, we quickly located the correct clinic and registered.

I had brought along a separate shirt on a hanger so

that I could change before seeing the doctor. It was still my belief that if I put on my best front, showed strength, and seemed not to be declining as rapidly as expected, then it would be more likely that the doctor would explore every other medical possibility.

After a short while, I was weighed, my blood pressure, pulse, and temperature were taken, and we were led to a small examining room. The nurse was very pleasant, and we thanked her for her kindness.

We had been in the small examining room about ten minutes, when there was a knock on the door, and Dr. H. entered the room with a pleasant smile on his face. He greeted us both, shook our hands, and said, "It's good to see you both again, and I am glad that I will be seeing you here on a regular basis."

When he finished his examination, he said, "You can get dressed now. I know that will help warm you up." The examining rooms always seemed to be cool, and when I would get undressed, it didn't take long for me start shivering. The chill would go right to my bones. Sometimes it would take hours before I would feel warm and comfortable. Wendy helped me get my socks, pants, and shirt on, and then I sat down in one of the chairs and slipped my feet into my shoes. During this time, the doctor was observing my movements, and after I was dressed, he asked, "Can you return in two weeks? There are some tests that I would like to schedule." "I can be here whenever you say!" I replied.

During my second visit to Dr. H., I underwent a series of nerve conduction tests, electromyography, similar to the ones I had in Wilmington. However, there were two doctors performing the tests this time, and the procedures required a much longer period of time than before. Also, the equipment seemed to be more sophisticated. I could hear the crackling sound as the needle was moved from one nerve group to another.

One of the doctors described the meaning of the modulations that were being produced, as well as the visual patterns displayed on a large, greenish screen. I didn't understand much of what the doctors were discussing, but I did get bits and pieces of the conversation, such as, "You can see the difference in this peak and the last one, which showed extensive abnormalities regarding this nerve group . . . Now, you see with this one there are abnormalities characteristic of anterior horn cell involvement and extensive nerve degeneration." The other doctor would respond from time to time to the comments of the doctor discussing the results. At several points during the tests, the doctor who seemed to be in charge would stop the procedure and indicate with his forefinger the areas on my body where fasciculations occurred.

Dr. H. met with me after the tests but said he would not have the final results that day. I seemed to feel very weak in the evenings but would feel stronger the next morning. This scenario bothered Dr. H., and he decided to try an additional test using a drug called Tensilon. After the injection of Tensilon, the doctor asked me to perform several activities that required my strength. Right after the injection and for maybe sixty seconds thereafter, I had a rush and felt stronger. The doctor seemed very pleased, and the other doctor, who always came in and examined me prior to Dr. H. seeing me, got very excited. In fact, it was the only time he had shown any kind of emotion whatsoever.

Dr. H. told me about a disease called myasthenia gravis, which had many symptoms that mimic ALS, but myasthenia gravis could be treated and was not considered to be terminal, resulting in death, as was ALS.

9

Dr. H. ordered special blood tests that could be fairly conclusive, regarding myasthenia gravis, but they returned with negative results. He also prescribed a drug called Mestinon, which I thought was helping, but after trying several different doses over a period of time, I experienced no real positive results. But Dr. H. did not give up. He had me examined and tested extensively by one of the leading authorities on myasthenia gravis in the country.

The results came up negative. I believe that Dr. H. wanted my disease not to be ALS so badly that he would not give up without covering every possibility. And that's what I wanted, too.

Dr. H. told me about a special treatment used with myasthenia gravis, called plasmapheresis, which was extremely effective but would require my staying in the hospital for two weeks. His question was, "Do you want to go through this very involved procedure?" My answer was, "I'm ready to try anything!" The arrangements were made, and I spent two weeks in the hospital having my blood drained, washed, and returned to my body in a continuous procedure, every other day, for the two-week period.

I had plenty of time on my hands to think during that two-week stay in the hospital. It wasn't pleasant to re-run, in my mind, the events of the last couple of months, and I certainly didn't want to think about what the future held for me. Also, the thought of Wendy and Amanda being left alone bothered me. What really bothered me was that I was not going to be with them anymore. I didn't want to die.

The only avenue that I had open, mentally, was to use my memory and travel back in time to more pleasant times in my life. I thought back to when Wendy and I had first met and started dating. We had some fantastic times together. But then I would see Wendy as she brought me to the hospital, and my mind would return to the present and all the problems that we faced.

I decided to travel further back in time. I was back in Washington, D.C., attending Woodrow Wilson High School. Those were great times filled with fond memories, and I had some wonderful friends. I would picture each of them in my mind and replay the fun times that we had together.

Life was simple back then. I liked school and was a good student with a fondness for sports. In addition to running track and playing football, I used to box at the local athletic club at our church.

My social life was particularly good. I was president of my high school fraternity, and every Friday night we would hold a meeting to handle important business such as raising funds to pay for our trip to Ocean City when school let out. After the meeting, there was always some place to go. Usually one or more of the sororities would have a party. The big decision to make was where to take your girlfriend on Saturday night.

Dating was an important part of my life in those days, and I made the most of it, dating different girls who were all very nice and lots of fun to be with. Generally, I would have a date for Friday night, one for Saturday night, and one at church youth group on Sunday evening.

During the summer months, there was always an embassy party or two each week, canoe trips on the Potomac to attend the outdoor concerts. There were plenty of parties at friends' homes and, of course, lots of good movies to see.

There was only one girl that I really became serious about, and it was her face that was now fixed in my mind. We spent a lot of time together and even went steady for a period of time. It always sounds ridiculous to adults to think that teenagers can know anything about love. And I felt the same way when my children were in their teens, but time has proven to me that it can happen. This girl was my first love, and my special feelings for her have lasted over many years. The sound of the door opening to my room brought me back to reality. It was dinner time and my tray had arrived.

We had completed the two weeks of plasmapheresis treatments. As with the Mestinon, I thought it was helping in the beginning, but it turned out to have no positive results. While I was in the hospital, I was also tested for temporomandibular joint syndrome (TMJ). This is an illness that produces many of the same symptoms that I experienced with my chewing and swallowing problems. The examination proved to be negative for TMJ.

Dr. H. was disappointed and, I believe, extremely frustrated at this point. Even the other doctor who had become so excited when I had the Tensilon test told me how sorry he was.

It was good to be back home with my family. Wendy

and Amanda had visited me regularly during the two weeks when I was in the hospital, and Amanda had made a large doll that she named Fred, so I would always have company and not get lonely. Fred sat in the large chair near the foot of my bed and remained there until I left the hospital.

Naturally, I was very disappointed that Dr. H.'s effort to uncover some disease other than ALS had not proven successful. No one likes to feel helpless, and my situation was leading to a feeling of being overwhelmed. Depression started to set in, and I knew that I had to put a stop to this draining feeling, because it would only make a very bad situation a whole lot worse.

I went back in time and read over all the research material that I had gathered about ALS. I studied every page of material searching for some sign of hope. Every time I found something that sounded as if it might have a possibility, I would make a copy of the material and send it to Dr. H., whom I was seeing only every two months at this point in time. I would receive a prompt and informative reply from Dr. H., explaining that he was already familiar with the information and that the research had turned out not to have any positive effect on ALS. But he always thanked me for whatever information I sent to him.

One day I discovered some research information that had just recently been published. It referred to a "lower form" of ALS. Officially, it was given the name multifocal motor neuropathy. Many of the symptoms, and the way they progressed over time, were quite similar to my own. The research and testing for this lower form of ALS had been carried out at the Department of Neurology at the University of Michigan. The doctors had used an immune suppressor called Cyclophosphamide, which had produced positive clinical improvement in the test patients.

I wrote to Dr. H. with all the details, and several days later he telephoned me. He was familiar with the research and agreed with my assessment that my illness did, in many ways, fit into the model of this lower ALS.

At my next appointment Dr. H. prescribed the drug Cytoxin for me to try for a short period of time, to see if we could get any positive results. This was a very powerful drug with possible bad side effects, some very serious. Dr. H. made arrangements for me to be seen every week in Salisbury to have blood tests and other lab procedures done. I hoped this would be the break I had been searching for. Maybe I didn't have to die!

Once again, we hit a dead end. After an appropriate period of time, Dr. H. discontinued my use of the drug. There had been no positive effects whatsoever, and I was approaching the time when continued use of the drug could be extremely hazardous. My condition continued to worsen, and Dr. H. admitted that he could not think of any other tests, procedures, or treatments to try.

Meanwhile, Wendy had found a regular part-time job, (twenty hours per week) after a long and frustrating search. My situation was such that I could not be left alone during the day because of the deterioration of my physical condition. I was unable to carry on simple daily activities. I was receiving home health care, which meant that a nurse came to my home twice a month, a physical therapist treated me every Tuesday and Thursday, and a nursing assistant stayed with me five days per week, until Wendy would arrive home in the afternoon from work.

At this point, I was seeing Dr. H. every two months. He was always a pleasure to see, but he was at a loss for anything new to try. He said that a number of my studies, including fasciculations, features on the electromyograph, and biopsies, showed abnormalities that were characteristic of ALS. Some of my clinical findings were also suggestive of ALS. And all the specific tests for myasthenia gravis had turned out negative. In one of his letters he wrote, "Again, I am sorry that I am not able to be more definite about what is going on. We will simply have to say you have ALS, and wait, and watch, and evaluate things as they develop."

Our living conditions in the small apartment were adding to what was already a bad situation for us, so we found a three-bedroom, two-bath brick home that rented for slightly less than what we were paying for the apartment. The house had a yard with plenty of trees and shrubs and a spot for some tomato plants and cucumbers. There were a large kitchen, lots of storage space, and a basement.

I soon found a favorite spot in the family room, which was actually part of the large kitchen. There was a large picture window that looked out on the back yard and beyond to a wooded area with trees and foliage. The couch was arranged so that I could sit next to the window and enjoy the beautiful view.

Moving to the house was something very special for all of us. We were starting to feel like real people again, and it made a tremendous difference in our family life. Amanda began to invite her friends from school to visit and play. Wendy put a bird feeder on the outside windowsill, next to where I sat on my end of the couch. Soon we had beautiful birds using the feeder, and I could watch them come and go. Nature is such a wondrous thing; whenever I would start to feel sorry for myself or get depressed, the sight of the multicolored birds, the lush green grass, and the large trees with their branches reaching out in every direction would help to calm my mind.

During this time, I wore a special brace that Dr. H. had the hospital design for me. The brace was padded and fit under my chin and along each side of my head. This upper support section was connected to metal support bars that were connected to a leather harness running from the back of my head to my lower back. The leather straps buckled around my chest. When I wore the brace, my head was held in a proper upright position. It was originally designed to enable me to sit up while riding in the car, but I found many other uses for it.

Also during this period, eating had become a labor-intensive process involving a considerable amount of time for each meal. Wendy prepared wonderful puréed items and each day would make up a lunch plate for me before she left for work. The nursing assistant would help me eat my lunch around 12:30 each day.

Even though I was growing weaker, Dr. H. was pleased that my arms and legs were still functioning, though I could not really participate in any meaningful physical activities. But most important, I was not experiencing much difficulty with my breathing. I still had to be very careful when I swallowed, and sometimes during the night I would wake up coughing, but those weren't really breathing problems. I had difficulty early on with breathing, and there was one incident after our move to Salisbury when I did end up in the hospital emergency room when my chest tightened.

My first neurologist in Wilmington had been right about my eating becoming a serious problem within six months, but thank goodness my breathing was not following the original prognosis!

10

As I looked out the window at the birds, I became fascinated by how they could maneuver by flapping their wings. It occurred to me that during the early history of aviation, humans built contraptions that mimicked the wing movement of the bird, but they all ended in failure. Humans finally settled for a fixed-wing device using auxiliary power. It occurred to me that we humans are intelligent but perhaps don't realize how limited we are when it comes to the wonders of nature. It was at this point in my life, while sitting there watching the wonders of nature, that I realized that I had made a terrible mistake! I had been counting on the doctors and medical science to fix my illness. I had not been listening. The doctor in Wilmington had told me there was nothing that could be done medically to stop this hideous disease or to heal me. The medical literature explained, in great detail, that there was no treatment and that ALS was a terminal disease. And Dr. H. had been up front with me, telling me that medical science didn't understand very much about ALS or exactly what ALS was.

I had been an entrepreneur all my life, or at least since age fourteen. I had started and operated many successful businesses over the years, and I had discovered at a very early age that if you really want to be sure that something is done right, you had better do it yourself.

What would I have done if someone had tried to take one of my businesses away from me? No way would I have just sat there and hoped someone would come along and help save me. I would have fought with every ounce of life that I had, and that is what I must do now—fight! There were certain truths that I had learned during my life, and I believed in them, and they had served me well: "Where there is a will there is a way." Though I had been told many times that old sayings are corny, I had based my whole life on them. I believed that the early bird would get the worm. I believed that right would win out over might. I believed that love was the energy of life. It was now time to really believe in myself.

That day, a large white envelope arrived in the mail. It was from an organization called the A.R.E., which was located in Virginia Beach, Virginia. I kept a metal letter opener handy, because the weakness in my right hand made it very difficult for me to open any type of mail. After several attempts, I was able to open one end of the large envelope.

Inside the envelope were numerous pieces of printed material, one of which was a letter explaining that my daughter, Debbie Atkinson, had given me a gift membership in the Association for Research and Enlightenment (A.R.E.). I read through some of the accompanying material, which explained details about the organization. As I continued to read, I came across the name Edgar Cayce, a name I was somewhat familiar with. I knew that he was reportedly a mystic or healer who had become famous for his ability to diagnose illnesses, and that at one time doctors from around the world had brought him their most difficult patients. I also knew he had died many years ago.

My first thought was to telephone my daughter and ask her why she had given me a membership in some organization involving mystics and hocus-pocus, but I realized that she was still at work.

Among the material in the envelope was a magazine called *Venture Inward.* It was quite attractive and contained beautiful pictures from nature. I started to read the magazine and found that some of the material was interesting and presented in a forthright manner, but some of the articles seemed to be foolishness about imaginary experiences. I wondered what connection my daughter had to this organization and why she thought I would be interested in being a member.

That evening I had my wife telephone Debbie. I told her about the material I had received from the A.R.E. and asked her why she had given me a gift membership in this organization and what connection she had with such a group. Debbie explained that she had been a member of the A.R.E. for a number of years but had never mentioned it to me because she knew that I would not understand nor accept the validity of Edgar Cayce and his work.

I was very surprised that she was involved with this group and asked her why she thought that I would want to be a member. She asked me if I had read any of the material and what I thought about it. "Well, I have read some of the stories in the magazine they sent and found some of them interesting, but some of them were really hard to believe," I answered.

Debbie said, "I have a book about Edgar Cayce that I want you to read. It's called *There Is a River.* It's a paperback, easy to read, and I believe you will find it to be extremely interesting. Let me bring it over. Read it as a favor to me." I asked her what it was about. Her answer was, "Please, just read it!"

Debbie brought the book by that evening, and I promised I would read it when I had time. That was a real laugh. Even though my time was running out, I wasn't putting the time that I had left to very good use.

The next morning, after the nurse's aide had bathed and dressed me, I was sitting upright with the help of my brace, preparing to be fed. I thought about Debbie, the A.R.E., and the book she had asked me to read. Later that afternoon, I decided to read some of the book to see why Debbie thought it was important.

I had the nurse's aide set up the wooden tray that fit over my lap and could be adjusted from a flat surface to several angles. She placed the book in front of me. I was right-handed but did not have much control with that hand anymore, so I turned the pages with my left hand.

At first, I thought the story was a little slow, but as I read on, it became very interesting, but more important the story started to sound real, as if it had actually taken place. My ability to read was hampered by the awkwardness of how I had to handle the book and by the fact that I tired very easily. It took me about three days to complete the book, but I must admit I did look forward to it each day, picking up where I had left off the day before.

If what I read in *There Is a River* was only half true, then Edgar Cayce was a remarkable man. I had to find out more about this man, so I began to research the information that I had read. It turned out that I was not the first skeptic who had decided to verify Edgar Cayce's legacy. Many independent researchers had done extensive documentation about the amazing life of this man. He had been investigated by major newspapers throughout his life, as well as by leading scientists and doctors.

There was so much irrefutable documentation available that I found myself confused. Being a very conservative hands-on type of person, I found it difficult to accept what I had learned. But the facts could not be denied. There was really something of substance to Edgar Cayce's ability to diagnose and recommend treatments for many individuals. I did not accept everything that Cayce expounded; some of it seemed too unbelievable.

Edgar Cayce had given thousands of medical readings, and many doctors from around the world, as well as very reputable doctors in this country, treated some of their most difficult patients with Cayce's assistance, and the results were remarkably successful.

By this point in time, Debbie and I had discussed the Cayce material extensively, and I asked her to find out if he had done a reading on ALS. The records indicated that there had been only one reading (5019-1) done on ALS, and Debbie got a copy of that reading from the A.R.E. library for me.

I was still very skeptical, but my medical condition was worsening, so I decided to read what Cayce had said about ALS: "Do the first things first. Begin with reading Exodus 19:5 and Deuteronomy 30. Apply these to self." While I had been quite active in the Episcopal church in my younger years, I hadn't been going to church regularly for twenty or more years and hadn't used prayer in I don't know how long. I had no real relationship with my Creator, and religion was not something that I spent much time thinking about. And when I saw that two of the recommendations in the Cayce reading involved reading Scripture, I said, "Now I know this is hocus-pocus." Yes, there was no question that Cayce had helped many sick individuals, as well as many doctors, but this was just too much for me to swallow. The reading was put up on the bookshelf, and that was the end of that foolishness for me.

I continued my boring daily routine. I was having a lot of difficulty with some of the personnel who were sent to my home by the home health agency. They were people who just wanted to put in their hours, to make some money. Their idea was that I needed a baby sitter, so they would check on me now and then but spent most of their time watching television, talking on the telephone, and raiding the refrigerator! After numerous complaints that went unheeded, I fired that particular health agency and found a new one that was much more professional and responsive to my needs.

As time passed, I knew that I had to do something or I wasn't going to live very long. I decided to read *There Is a River* again. That night a strange feeling came over me, and out of the blue I prayed, asking, "What should I do?" Then I took my sleeping pills and dozed off.

It had been a long time since I had had a dream, at least one that I remembered, but that night I had a very vivid dream. In my dream a group of doctors were discussing ALS research. None of them could agree on any aspect of the disease or how they should proceed. Suddenly, a large door slammed shut, and I was in a room, alone, sitting at a desk. I was reading *There Is a River.* The next morning I remembered exactly what had happened in that dream; in fact, the drama continued to play over and over, even when I was being bathed and fed breakfast.

Immediately after eating, I had the nurse's aide help me move over to my special seat next to the window. She attached and adjusted my head brace so that I could hold my head in an upright position. As she started back to the kitchen area, I said, "Please hand me those papers on the shelf," and I pointed with my left thumb to the Cayce reading. I read the material over several times that morning and again that afternoon. It just didn't make sense to me. Why was it so specific about little incidental things such as a special combination of oils to be used during the massage portion of the treatment? What was a wet cell? I just didn't feel comfortable with what I was reading.

I called to the nurse, who was filling out some paperwork, and asked, "Would you please come here? I need your help." She came over to where I was sitting and started to reach toward my lap tray. She must have thought I wanted her to help me to the bathroom. I said, "No, I don't need to get up. I would like you to hand me that Bible on the top shelf of the bookcase." She got the Bible and put it on my reading tray. I had decided to read the two Scriptures that were mentioned in the reading. I was curious to see what they said and what connection they could possible have to my illness.

Exodus 19:5 consisted of several sentences, but there was nothing there that said anything about illness. So I turned to Deuteronomy 30. It was like being hit in the face with a brick, because it's where Moses tells, point-blank, how to have good health and live or how to be sick and die.

He doesn't mince words in Deuteronomy 30. And it struck me so powerfully that I read it over and over again. When Wendy came home from work, I asked her to sit on the couch with me. We read it together, and we discussed it, and then we read it again. I said, "Let's find a church and check it out!" I had read an article in *Venture Inward* magazine about how to pray, and I started following those instructions. I never prayed for a miracle or asked to be healed—only to develop a relationship with my Creator so that I could once again feel comfortable and know Him. How could I expect help when I had been too busy, wrapped up in my own little world?

As my relationship advanced, I became comfortable praying for guidance and intuitiveness to know what I could do to help myself. Little did I know the chain of amazing events that were to take place in my life because of what Debbie had set in motion with her gift to me!

Wendy and I started to check out the local churches. We wanted a church that had a good Sunday school and youth program, for Amanda's benefit. We picked the First Presbyterian Church in Salisbury. The Cayce reading returned me to God, it returned me to prayer, and it returned me to church. And from that point on, my prayer always ended with "Lord, guide me, direct me to those people, places, and things that will help me to help myself to be healthy and strong physically, mentally, and spiritually." I never prayed for a miraculous healing or a cure. I have prayed only for the guidance and the intuitiveness to know what I can do to help myself and to know how my relationship with my Creator can be strengthened.

Seeing how that part of the reading had turned out to be positive in my life, I decided to follow the rest of the reading, which I really considered far-out. It was at this point in time that I first had contact with Bruce Baar, a young man who had dedicated his life to study Edgar Cayce and his health readings. Bruce manufactured many of the devices that Cayce recommended to treat numerous types of serious illnesses. Bruce did not make any medical claims about the devices, but he believed in the Edgar Cayce readings and truly wanted to help people. He and his wife Kathy turned out to be real friends to me and my family.

After meeting and talking with many members of the A.R.E. from all around the world and hearing how they had been helped by following many of the Cayce readings over the years, I felt much better about my decision to try to help myself. I didn't have a lot to lose because the medical community had already told me there was no known cause or treatment for ALS.

A wonderful experience that boosted my spirit was

when I met Dr. C. Norman Shealy. Dr. Shealy is a neuro-surgeon and psychologist whom I met through my involvement with the A.R.E. I discussed with him my diagnosis of ALS and the fact that I had decided to follow the Cayce reading and supplement my traditional medical treatment with those alternative treatments that I could believe in.

Dr. Shealy is a soft-spoken man, yet while in his presence, I felt a powerful energy of compassion. His advice was for me to follow whatever recommendations that my neurologist had, regarding medical treatment, but he believed very much that hope and one's will to overcome illness could sometimes lead to miraculous events.

Dr. Shealy is the founder of the Shealy Institute in Springfield, Missouri, a center for health care and pain and stress management. He has authored a number of books including *The Pain Game* and *The Creation of Health.*

My wet cell unit, which Cayce had recommended for treatment of ALS, arrived from Bruce Baar, and I started following the regimen, which included a massage every day.

The wet cell appliance produces a small but measurable electrical current that, according to Cayce, can be used to stimulate the growth of nerve tissue and balance the glandular system. The wet cell was most often recommended for incoordination between the sympathetic and cerebrospinal nervous systems.

Modern medicine today has incorporated the use of microcurrent electric stimulation into the field of energy medicine as an innovative medical paradigm based on physics instead of chemistry. The study of the body's physics was pioneered by Dr. Robert O. Becker, M.D., who spent more than thirty years developing theories that an electromagnetic field is the basis to all life processes, something that Cayce indicated by recommending the use of the wet cell in nearly 100 readings for more than 150 different ailments.

After three months my condition was still getting worse. After six months I was very frustrated, because nothing was happening. I called Bruce to see if I might be using the device incorrectly. I went over my daily routine step by step with Bruce. He verified that I was following the reading correctly, but reminded me that the reading said, "One must be consistent and persistent." I had talked to Bruce many times over the months, and he always took time to be very pleasant and helpful, and if I was feeling down, he would try to pick my spirits up and make me feel good.

I considered my options. I had the Cayce reading and was doing whatever I could to help myself, and I had what the medical community offered: no hope! So it seemed to me that my choice was pretty clear. The Cayce material provided me with a focus, a door that opened up to hope. I decided to choose hope and continued the Cayce treatment. In retrospect, I had expected too much too fast. When I said at the end of six months that nothing was happening, I had failed to notice that I was still alive!

I used my special prayer regularly and started to receive guidance. Sometimes it came in the form of a dream. Other times I would be aware of a warm and exciting presence around me, and I would receive the guidance I was seeking. This warm, exciting feeling was not new to me, but it had been many years since I had experienced it.

As a young boy growing up in Washington, D.C., I spent much of my time in and around the construction site of the Washington National Cathedral. During summer break from school, I would be at the Cathedral almost every day. It was my special place to go to meet new and interesting friends, such as the stone masons who cut by hand and fitted each section of stone together. There were artisans who would start with a large slab of stone and, using special tools, would create beautiful designs and statues that were raised by large construction cranes to help form the walls and columns of the Cathedral.

The construction workers were nice, and they would talk to me about the special underground tunnels and secret passageways, some of which had stairways that were inside the large walls leading from the many different chapels up to the many balconies, and some to the roof hundreds of feet above.

The Cathedral was about half completed at this point in time, and many of the chapels had beautifully carved altars, as well as magnificent murals. I would kneel at the different altars and pretend I could see God there, and I would talk with Him about the things I liked to do, about the construction work being done, and why it was taking so many years to build the Cathedral. I asked Him why my father had been sick for such a long time and why he had to die.

All of a sudden my memory focused on my Father. I was ten years old when he died. He had been ill, off and on, for a number of years. During his last year, he had nurses with him around the clock at our home. There were times when he would be taken to the hospital and then several days later returned home by ambulance. I rarely saw him other than to say good night, and then many times he was asleep. My mother told me that he had high blood pressure and had suffered several heart attacks.

I have very few memories of my father and me doing things together, but there is one time that stands out in my mind. It was a Sunday, and my father was listening to the radio in the sun parlor of our home in Washington, D.C. I was sitting on the floor next to his chair. My mother, who was teaching Sunday school, had not returned home yet, and I don't remember where my older brother was at the time.

Suddenly, the radio program was interrupted by a special news broadcast—the Japanese had attacked the United States and bombed Pearl Harbor.

My father jumped to his feet. I hadn't seen him move that fast before, and I had never seen him really excited until that moment. He reached down, took my hand, and said, "Son, we are going for a ride." I had never been in the car alone with my father, never just him and me.

He quickly led me through the living room, then down the hall to the kitchen, where he plucked the car keys from the key rack and told our cook, Fanny, about the radio report. He said, "I am going to the Embassy," and out the door we went.

Our family had two cars—one was a two-door roadster convertible my mother drove, and the other was what I called the big car, a four-door Packard sedan. My father opened the door to the big car and lifted me onto the seat and closed the door. Then he went around to the driver's side and got in the car, and we were on our way.

He drove out of our driveway and down 38th Street three blocks to Massachusetts Avenue, where he turned left. We drove fast down Massachusetts Avenue. I stood on the floor, holding on to the dashboard so that I could see out through the windshield. I had never been allowed to stand up while the car was moving.

Very soon, we had to stop because there were a lot of policemen in the street, holding back a large crowd of excited people.

My father drove our car around two other cars and right up to where the policemen were standing. Then he sounded the car horn several times until one of the policemen came over to talk to him. The policeman said,

"You can't pass this point. All people are banned from this area." My father reached inside his coat pocket and brought out his brown leather billfold with its gold badge on the inside flap.

I had seen my father's gold badge many times before, as he was an official with the city government. He showed the gold badge to the policeman and said, "Have them clear the way for my car all the way to the Embassy driveway." The policeman ran over to several other policemen and talked to them. Then they opened a pathway through the police lines, and we dove right up to the entrance and stopped next to a big red fire engine and a red fire chief's car.

When the fire chief saw my father, he got out of his car and rushed over to talk with him. By the way he greeted my father, I knew they must be friends. I heard the fire chief say, "The G-men won't let us go in, even with all that smoke pouring out of those upper windows," and he pointed at the Embassy. He said, "They are burning all their secret papers, and we can't do a thing about it. They have even refused permission for my men to enter the grounds." The fire chief looked angry. My father asked, "Are they claiming diplomatic immunity?" "Yes, they are," he answered, "and according to the G-men, we have to honor their immunity even though they've bombed our ships and killed hundreds of our sailors. It doesn't make any sense to me!"

That was my big day with my father. At the time, I didn't understand anything about what was going on. I just knew that I was with my father and it was an exciting time for me.

It is amazing how one's mind can, all of a sudden, produce an event from so long ago and with so much detail. These thoughts of my father, of the few clear and meaningful memories, became a source of strength for me.

Now my thoughts were drifting back to the Cathedral

and my conversation with God about why my father died. I didn't get an answer to my question, so I just thought about the Cathedral. I had two favorite altars out of the many that had already been constructed.

One was the large central altar for the main floor of the Cathedral. I used to crawl under the prayer-rail rope. That rope was magnificent. It was made from large twisted strands that were dark red in color, and it felt smooth like velvet. At each end of the rope were large gold tassels. I was always very careful whenever I crawled under the altar rope, because one time I had caused it to fall to the floor and had a difficult time getting it back in place.

Once I had crawled under the rope, I could stand close to the altar and touch it with my hands. It was so high that I couldn't see all the way to the top. I liked to put both my hands against the limestone surface and think about heaven.

But my number-one favorite altar was located in the small children's chapel. There was a special kneeling cushion in that chapel. It ran the entire length of the altar rail and had wonderful scenes portraying Noah's ark and all the different animals. Many times I would talk to God for a while and then would lie down on the beautiful cushion and take a nap. I would dream about heaven and angels and David and Goliath and stories from the Bible that I had heard about in Sunday school.

Not every time, but many times, God would answer my questions when I was in the children's chapel. He didn't speak to me when He answered my questions—I didn't hear His voice—but I knew that He was there with me. There was a special warm and exciting feeling in and around my body, and somehow I would just know that the thoughts that were in my mind, at that time, were His answers to my questions, I just knew it.

Now, so many years later, I was having conversations

with God in the same way that I did when I was a young boy in the Cathedral. My thoughts were telling me that I had to use my mind to heal my relationship with God first, before I could hope to heal my body. I understood more clearly what Edgar Cayce had meant in the reading when he said, "First things first!"

I was becoming a firm believer in the blending of modern technology and ancient wisdom. The importance of self-reliance, combining traditional medicine and the healing energy from within, became my foundation.

My spirit was lifted, and the time I had spent on the Cayce treatment was working. I had been looking for physical signs of healing and had overlooked what had been taking place spiritually. Cayce was right when he spoke about a belief in oneness. We are whole beings, not separate parts made up of a body, a mind, and a soul. If I were going to live, I would have to be healthy as a whole human being.

That night, I said prayers of thanks. How wonderful it was to be back on speaking terms with God again!

11

The A.R.E. had vast amounts of information about meditation, visualization, and guided imagery, and I began to study these subjects. I also started using the VCR to tape segments of programs from television shows that documented true stories about people who had been able to overcome serious injuries and illnesses.

Every day, I watched my videotape and used the wet cell, massage, meditation, and visualization. I prayed my special prayer and developed guided healing imagery.

Positive energy flowed through me and around me. My awareness was raised, and after almost ten months, I realized that my physical condition had leveled off. I had been so intent on watching for something spectacular to happen that I had overlooked the fact that my symptoms weren't getting any worse.

That was an exciting time for me. My energy level went up, and I spent a lot more time using my guided healing imagery. Before, I had been doing it once a day; now I was doing it two and sometimes three times a day.

When I watched the videotape, I used to say I wanted to be like those people. Now when I watched the tape, I said I am going to do what they have done. I am going to get well and beat this disease. Before, I was saying it to myself in my mind; now I was saying it out loud in a strong, firm voice. I really believed that I could do it.

Several days later, after having finished my wet cell treatment, the physical therapist arrived. He came twice a week and was very familiar with the wet cell unit. In fact, when he first started working with me, he was so interested in the wet cell and the Cayce readings that he drove up to Virginia Beach and spent two days at the A.R.E. talking with people and researching the readings about other illnesses that he was working with.

Now he was disconnecting the attachments from the wet cell unit and was helping me roll over from my back to my stomach so that he could start the massage. On the days that the physical therapist came, he would complete the physical therapy treatment and then do the massage.

Suddenly, I realized that I was holding my head up as he turned me over. Of course, the first thing I did was to lay my head down on the bed, because I knew that I wasn't supposed to be able to hold my head up. I was in shock and not really sure what was going on.

The impact of what had just happened started to set in. I immediately lifted my head again and held it up. I could really do it! I could move my head up and down! I repeated the movement over and over again. I got very excited, and so did the physical therapist. I was laughing and filled with excitement. He completed the massage and asked me to see if I could still move my head. I could, but my neck was starting to feel weak, so he told me to take it easy and not overdo it.

I was so excited I could hardly wait for Wendy to come

home. Just as soon as we heard her come into the house, the physical therapist, who had decided to stay for a while, went to get Wendy and brought her back to the bedroom. I showed her how I could lift my head. We both held on to one another and laughed and cried.

As each day passed, my routine became more exciting, because I could see and feel the improvements that were taking place. I was now able to sit up and hold my head up on my own, with no more need for the brace. I was regaining my strength and the mobility in my arms, especially my right arm and hand. I still needed help to get up off the couch or out of a chair, but once I was up, I could stand and walk on my own. I was still a little off balance, and every now and then I would have to lean against the wall or hold onto the back of a chair to balance myself, but I could walk and hold my head up.

Be "consistent and persistent." Those words from the Cayce reading were etched in my mind, and I continued my daily treatments. In fact, I increased the amount of time that I spent on visualization and watching the videotape, and I had already increased the number of times that I was doing my guided healing imagery. I thanked God for answering my prayers by guiding me to those people, places, and things that could help me to help myself.

I had to continue to use a special shower chair, but I could bath myself at this point and, with some difficulty, dress myself. Reaching up with my arms and hands to wash my hair was still extremely difficult, so I still needed help with some things. But I was definitely on my way, once again, to being a functioning human being.

There were days when I tried too much and would wash out and have a very low energy level. Every so often I would have a little setback, but I continued to improve, and it was glorious.

At this point in time, I was seeing Dr. H. about every six months, but for some reason it had been seven or maybe eight months since I had been to the clinic in Chapel Hill. Dr. H. was pleased and impressed with my overall improvement—especially with the fact that I was able to hold my head up with no difficulty. He hadn't seen me at my worst, so he didn't realize how drastic the change really was.

I had never discussed with Dr. H. the Cayce reading or any of the other alternative treatments that I had been doing at home. So I decided to tell him about some of the things, though I never mentioned Edgar Cayce. After all, this was a teaching hospital, and I don't think Dr. H. would have accepted the sort of alternative modalities that I had been using, as having any therapeutic value.

During our discussion he did say, "Whatever you are doing seems to be good for you, so continue the good work." I think his scientific mind was in control at that point and he was questioning my improvement. He had seen all the traditional symptoms of ALS that had developed. He had seen the results from all the EMGs. He had proven without any doubt that I didn't have myasthenia gravis. Also, he was the one who personally did the muscle and nerve biopsies.

As he is a medical doctor and a scientist, his belief system was based on what he had learned over the years through practical experience. So I can imagine the conflict that was going on within his cognitive process. He scheduled my next appointment for six months, so Wendy and I headed back to Salisbury. I followed my program diligently and continued to improve.

During the next several months, I was able to reverse almost every debilitating symptom that I had! I was able to hold my head in a proper upright position, I was able to lift my arms over my head, I could brush my teeth, and I could comb my hair. I could shower on my own, dress myself, and walk around and up and down steps without any assistance. I was still having some problems with my balance, but I was very careful.

By the end of the fourteenth month from the day that I had started to use the wet cell, I had reversed all the symptoms that I had suffered and struggled with during my illness, except for two. My palate was still paralyzed and not functioning at all, and I had very little use of the little finger on my right hand.

I had beaten the odds just like the people who were on the videotape that I watched regularly for inspiration and hope. I had watched that tape hundreds of times during my illness, trying to identify with each person who had overcome his or her terminal condition, and now I had become one of them. In addition my fear about dying was gone. It really hadn't bothered me for some time, because once I put together the healing program, my mind was occupied with positive images and self-talk.

After approximately twelve months of being on a liquid purée feeding regimen, once again I could eat, chew, and swallow all the solid foods that I had missed so much during my illness. But I did not regain the ability to chew and swallow regular food when my other symptoms reversed. I had tried on several occasions to chew and swallow but was unable to do so.

How did I get to the point of being able to eat again? Wendy had driven me up to an area in the North Carolina mountains to meet with Dr. Harvey Bank (Ph.D. in biophysics and chemistry). Harvey had left his research and teaching position at a medical school and was working directly with individuals. He had helped people who had differing physical problems, and I thought maybe he could do something about my swallowing and the fact that my palate was still paralyzed.

After about an hour of bodywork Harvey said, "I'm

sorry, but I can't do anything for your palate." I was very disappointed. I looked at Wendy and said, "Well, I guess it was too much to expect that I would be able to eat real food again." Without hesitating, Harvey said, "I can fix that right now!" He did something under my jaw and then to my throat and neck. When he finished, he said, "You can go out right now and have a roast beef dinner, vegetables, salad—eat anything you want."

Wendy walked across the room and stood next to me, both of us in disbelief. But he was convincing, and he hadn't said, "Maybe this will work." He had said, "You can now eat solid food."

My oldest son, Michael, owned a restaurant in the mountains nearby in a little town called Banner Elk. I asked Wendy to drive me over to Mike's restaurant, and off we went. After we arrived there, I ordered prime rib, mashed potatoes, green beans, and a salad. Mike looked at me and said, "What are you going to do with that?" My answer was quick and to the point: "I'm going to eat it." He was shocked.

I wasn't convinced yet that I could do it, but I was going to try. The waiter brought the meal, and I cleaned my plate. I had no problem chewing or swallowing, which was an unbelievable feeling, and I have been eating ever since. There are people who have suggested that when my other symptoms reversed I was actually capable of eating at that time but had a mental block and all Harvey did was give me permission to believe that I could eat.

Whether Harvey physically changed something or emotionally changed something, I don't know and I don't care. There was a time in my life when I believed I needed to understand the reason for everything that happened, but now my feelings are that it would be nice to have all the answers, but I can accept and experience good things happening in my life without having to understand why. Remember, I had always been a very conservative person, and I had fought against the Cayce therapies in the beginning. I wasn't that thrilled with the wet cell unit in the beginning. And an exact mixture of three oils for the massage didn't make any sense to me at all.

What I did learn, because of my illness, was that I wasn't nearly as smart as I thought I was nor was the medical community. I changed my perspective regarding what I thought must be and what I believed would be. My awareness was raised considerably, and my thought process was freed from years of outdated and erroneous information that had become part of my belief system. I now have an open mind! What a powerful instrument an open mind can be.

Having an open mind doesn't mean that I accept every quack idea that comes along, but what it does mean is that I no longer judge people. I listen to what they have to say, no matter how far-out it is, and then I either find it acceptable or unacceptable for me. The very things that I used to save my life would be considered very strange and unacceptable to many people. But that is their problem, not mine!

After I got my diet straightened out, I felt much better. Emotionally I was much stronger, spiritually I was even stronger, and physically I was doing great!

From that point on, I decided to take charge of my own health care. I searched out doctors that fit into my wellness plan and formed a support team. But I was the captain, and the final decisions were mine to make. The team consisted of—first and foremost—my family, a general family physician to take care of my basic health needs, and Dr. H. for my ALS. He had always shown deep and sincere concern for me not only as a patient but also as a human being. I found a fantastic psychiatrist to help with my mental health and to treat my sleeping problem. I also consulted a very intuitive doctor whose specialty is rheumatology. He treats the arthritis that had developed in my joints because of my lack of proper exercise during the time when I was in bad shape. Finally, I have my church and my prayer sessions with God for my spiritual health.

I put this support team together myself, and I am in complete charge of my wellness program and my health care. One should never give up the authority or personal responsibility for his or her own health care. To do so is to feel helpless, and that only makes a bad situation worse.

Even though I wasn't up to full speed yet and knew it was going to take some time, I felt the need to be doing something productive with my time. So I started a mind-body study and support group in Salisbury. The group is open to the general public, and there are no fees required to be a member. Members of the group are local people who are interested in exploring the mind-body connection. Some members are suffering from a particular illness, and others just want to learn more about wellness.

We meet every other week. I try to motivate members and get them interested in how to use the subconscious mind to help control the mechanisms they have within them to maintain their health and to develop a positive attitude. We learn about proper breathing, good nutrition, exercise, massage, and many other wellness techniques. Each member knows that if he or she needs emotional support, the group will be there to help.

I was feeling good, and having been an entrepreneur most of my adult life, I decided it was time to get back into business and make some money. It would be nice to be a financially contributing member of the family again. But what kind of business could I start with no money? It would have to be something that didn't require any equipment or employees, and I would need to be able to run it from our house.

As I tried to come up with some ideas about what kind of business fit my criteria, I remembered my "To Do File." Over the years, I would come up with new and interesting ideas, so I developed a file to store literature and information in. But after everything that we had been through—moving from Wilmington to Salisbury and then moving twice since then—I had no idea were the file might be or even if we might still have it.

The search began for the file in the many boxes filled with old tax returns and papers from businesses I had previously owned. There were old family records, photos, and lots of Father's Day cards and birthday cards from over the years. It took me weeks to sort through all those storage boxes. Each time I would find something that was really interesting, I would stop and read it, and wonderful memories would flood into my mind. It was a very slow process, but I had plenty of time, and I was really enjoying myself.

Finally, there it was—a bulging manila envelope with "To Do File" written in large red letters. I spent several days sorting through all the material I had put away. There were numerous ideas to choose from, such as fish farming, board games, panning for gold, a special line of clothing for handicapped people, a specialty line of suntan lotion, and many, many more, but everything that I looked at required some kind of resources and money.

"Be persistent." It had worked before, so I kept looking until I found an idea that really interested me, and it was something I could do on my own from the house and required very little money to get started. I decided to publish a magazine! Salisbury didn't have a local magazine, and I thought this might work. There was no competition, it was something that the community needed, and it was a project I could handle on my own.

The library was the place to start. I spent several weeks

reading books and magazine articles about how to get into the publishing business—more particularly, how to start and develop a magazine. First, I had to come up with a good name that would attract attention. I decided on *American Lifestyles—Salisbury/Rowan.* Salisbury was the city, and Rowan was the county. And *American Lifestyles* was an eye catcher. I put together a mock-up, then designed a good cover and used pages from various other magazines, so that I could show potential advertisers what the magazine would look like. There were blank pages that indicated the different sized advertisements available, as well as a rate card showing the cost for each ad size based upon how many months the ad was to run.

I would be selling ad space to local merchants, businesses, organizations, and anyone else that I might think of who could benefit from this type of exposure. The idea was to sell enough advertising space and collect enough money in advance to have the first issue of the magazine printed. I had already figured out a unique way to distribute the magazine and develop a large readership base immediately. I would place the magazine in every doctor's and dentist's waiting room, free of charge. Also, I would place the magazine in waiting rooms at our two local hospitals, as well as in all the medical clinics and labs.

If it were free, I knew they would have no objection to having the magazine in their waiting rooms, and what do people do in waiting rooms? They read magazines!

The first day I started calling on potential advertisers, I sold space to every merchant whom I visited, a total of six sales. All six sales were for a twelve-month period, and I collected the first month's payment in advance. One of those six ads was for a full page, and I negotiated a discount in return for an advance payment equal to the cost of the ad for six months.

I found that almost everyone liked the idea, and selling ad space was not difficult. It wasn't long until I had raised the financial resources to pay for the first printing. Wendy and I had designed the layout, and I was off to see the printer.

The first issue was published, and it was a hit. I wrote the editorial and some of the articles. I got two local colleges to write monthly articles as a public service. I had Amanda write a kid's column. Wendy wrote several articles. A friend of Wendy's, Helen, wrote a column about microwave cooking. I interviewed the sheriff, and he wrote a great article about the responsibilities of the sheriff's department. I asked the daughter of a friend from church, Blake, to write a teen column, and I found a friend from church, Robin, who had a degree in journalism and became the feature writer. Then I bought some material from a company who specializes in supplying magazines with general interest articles.

Things were moving right along, and I had already started making plans to start magazines in other communities. It was too good to be true! But, once again, I had to face disaster. The magazine was going very well, but I was moving too fast. There was plenty of healing that still needed to take place in my body, and I had been so busy with the magazine that I had stopped doing all the healthy things that I should. I had also stopped listening to my body and its needs. It became very clear that the magazine venture was too stressful, and my health started to suffer, and some of my old symptoms started to reappear. I became very anxious, and then depression started to set in.

I was very disappointed. This was my chance to take my place as a productive member of the family once again and relieve some of the heavy financial burden that Wendy had been carrying. But Wendy was the first person to see the negative effect that the stress was having on me, and she made herself quite clear: "I'm not going to watch you jeopardize all the hard work that we have put into your recovery." She was absolutely right.

It was difficult for me to let go of something special that I had created, but there was no choice. I had to leave the magazine business, so I turned it over to Robin, my feature writer.

Emotionally, I felt as if I were letting my family down, and depression really set in. It was time to put my wellness plan into action and call upon the team member who was best equipped to help me help myself. Quickly, I telephoned the psychiatrist on my team and set up an appointment. Wendy and I met with him the first time and explained what the basic problem was. After that, I saw him about three or four times.

He helped me understand my limitations, as well as my role in life regarding my family. What was important to the family was that I stay alive, and what I had to offer was of much greater value than earning money. After about three months of meditation, visualization, and a new guided imagery, the depression was gone, and I was back on track. I had to understand my role in the family as well as my role in life.

After getting out from under the stress of the magazine, my health improved. Still, I needed something to do with my time. It was necessary for me find some way of feeling productive yet at the same time keep my stress under control and allow the healing to continue. I knew at that point that my working days were over; my nervous system had been through too much.

I joined the Thursday morning men's prayer group at church. We would meet at 6:30 a.m. Some of the members were retired, but most were men who stopped by on their way to work. We prayed for people who were experiencing difficulties in their lives, and we prayed for our community, our country, and all world leaders.

It was at this men's prayer group that I met one of the kindest and most loving people I have ever known. Mort Rochelle was his name, and he had a tremendous capacity to love people. Knowing him had a wonderful impact on my life, as well as on the lives of many others, young and old.

Mort developed cancer, and his body died quickly, but I know his spirit lives on. I pray, quite often, that among the many assignments that our Creator has for Mort, one of them will be to act as a guardian angel for me and my family. I miss Mort so very much that I find it difficult to return to the prayer group.

I volunteer at our local homeless shelter and soup kitchen. So do Wendy and Amanda. I have discovered that every time I help someone else, I am helping myself grow stronger and healthier, not only physically but spiritually, as well.

My life was moving along very well, and I had more appreciation for all the wonderful people around me, as well as the wonders of nature. I remember reading an article about nature and how it can be good for one's health. "The roar of the surf, the solitude of the woods, or the grandeur of the mountains can improve everybody's health," experts say. According to health psychologist Steven Tovian, Ph.D., of Evanston Hospital in Illinois, "studies show looking at and being in beautiful places slows one's heart rate and may also give the immune system a boost." It was a very special time for me, and I was thankful to be alive and to be able to love and be loved.

Things were good for Wendy, Amanda, and me. Wendy had turned a part-time job into a full-time position that she really enjoyed. Amanda was growing into a fine young lady, and she was an excellent student. Amanda also excelled at athletics, and she brought much joy and happiness into my life. We didn't have a lot of tangible wealth, but what we did have was of greater value than I could have ever hoped for in life. We had each other's love and caring.

Yes, things were moving along quite smoothly. But little did I know what was in store for me. My life was about to change dramatically.

12

The telephone rang one evening while I was watching the news on television. A female's voice weakly asked, "Can I speak to David Atkinson?" I answered, "This is David Atkinson." There was silence. After pausing for a few seconds, I once again said, "Hello, this is David Atkinson." The voice on the telephone asked, "Is this the David Atkinson who had ALS and cured himself?" I was taken aback by the question, and now the silence was on my part. Finally, I gained my composure and said, "I do have ALS, and I have been able to reverse most of the major symptoms that were stopping me from living a reasonably normal life."

The lady on the telephone identified herself and followed by saying, "My husband has been diagnosed with ALS, and we just today received a confirmation of the diagnosis from Duke Medical Center." She went on to explain that her husband had been told by a local neurologist and then by doctors at Duke that there was no known cause of ALS and that at this time there is no treatment for the disease. She and her husband had read all the literature and had been told that ALS is a terminal illness and perhaps he might have two to three years of progression before death.

Her voice was now very weak, and I could hear the emotional strain when she said, "As my husband and I were leaving the clinic area, one of the nurses who had been present off and on during our visit approached me and handed me a piece of folded paper." She said, "Please don't tell anyone that I gave this to you, and please wait until you're outside before you read this note."

It turned out that the note gave my name and phone number and explained that a friend, who is also a nurse, had heard about my recovery and had reported all the details to this nurse. The note ended by saying, "Maybe this man will have some answers for you."

We talked at length, and I tried to answer her questions, but I was really uncomfortable with this situation that I found myself in. Now her voice was stronger and less emotional, "Will you meet with my husband and me, so we can talk some more?" She continued, "We don't live too far from Salisbury and would like to meet you and see if you can help us!" My reply was slow, and now I was feeling a swell of emotion in my throat as I said, "I'm not sure what I can do to help your husband." The woman said, "Please, just meet with us and talk about what you did to overcome your ALS. Please, it would mean so very much to both of us!"

I agreed to meet with them in the lobby of the local Holiday Inn. There was plenty of seating area in the lobby, especially on the upper level, where we would have privacy. The rest of that evening I felt apprehensive as I discussed with Wendy the details of the phone call and the fact that I would be meeting with these strangers tomorrow morning at 9:30. Wendy didn't seem to be disturbed about what I had agreed to and said, "Perhaps you can help in some way. Don't worry about it; just re-lax, and it will work out fine."

The next morning, I arrived a half hour early. I wanted to have a chance to relax and think about what I was go-ing to say. What would they think about the alternative therapies that I had used? Would they think that I was weird and out of touch with reality? Or would they be open to a different approach of dealing with a serious illness?

They arrived at 9:20 a.m. and we began to talk. There were many questions. They wanted to know everything about my condition, how it started, and exactly how I reversed it. We lost track of time as I attempted to ex-plain about my personal healing program. It was very difficult for me to explain everything so that they could understand exactly what I was talking about. It was all very clear in my mind—I knew exactly what I needed to say—but it wasn't easy for me to put my thoughts into words.

I glanced at my watch. It was almost 2:00 p.m. They must have noticed that I looked at my watch, because they both did the same thing. Mrs. S. spoke up, "We have talked right through lunch. I can't believe that we have been talking nonstop for over four-and-a-half hours." She looked at me and said, "You must be hungry. Can we buy you lunch?" Then Mr. S. said, "Yes, please, let's have lunch together!" It was too late to eat at the hotel, be-cause the dining room had closed. And I needed some time to relax and think about what was happening. I said, "Thank you, but I'm really not hungry. Maybe if we get together again we can have lunch." Without hesita-tion Mr. S. broke in, "Do you have to go now? There is so much more that we want to know. Can you stay until 3:00 p.m.?" It was 4:30 before we parted that day, and we did see each other again. In fact, we visited together numer-ous times.

Over the next couple of weeks, I received other telephone calls from people who had been diagnosed with ALS and had heard about me. Two of the ladies in the mind-body support group asked me to meet with them individually and help them set up a self-care wellness program.

Then a couple of newspaper articles were written about what I had been able to accomplish. Next came several magazine articles, one of which was an in-depth feature article about how I was "Winning over Lou Gehrig's Disease." By this point in time, I was hearing from so many people that I couldn't talk with them in detail, because there wasn't enough time. We had call-waiting service on our telephone, and I would have to put someone from Florida on hold to answer a call from someone in New York, Texas, or California. Also during this time period, several more ALS people came to see me in Salisbury to seek my help. These were people who came from other states.

It became obvious that I had to get control of the situation. "First things first," is what the readings said. I prayed several times each day, first giving thanks for the many blessings I had received so far during my life. I had come to understand how fortunate I had been over the years. I really had received much more than my lifestyle had deserved.

Next, I prayed for guidance about how I could help these people who were turning to me and looking for answers. These were people who were in crisis, who were desperate, and who had been—in many cases—discarded by the medical community. Some of the statements made to these people by physicians and other health care professionals had virtually preprogrammed them to self-destruct.

Even though it had been happening for a while, I still found it wondrous to receive direct answers to specific questions I would ask during my prayers. Sometimes I would receive answers in vivid, detailed dreams. Other times I would have a "knowing." I would be aware of a presence all around me, accompanied by a warm feeling, and the answer would appear in my thought process just as it had when I was a young boy in the children's chapel at the Cathedral.

I became aware that I needed to put together a booklet describing the different modalities I had used and an explanation about how they worked. But each time I tried to put information into a written form, I ended up with pages and pages of material that many times was hard for me to follow. So how could I hope to make it clear enough for others to understand?

The answer came to me in a dream. In the dream, I was going through the boxes I used to store all the material I had gathered during my illness. Each time I found material that explained meditation, visualization, guided imagery, healing music, the wet cell, massage, nutrition, supplements, antioxidants, or any other supportive material, I would lay it on the floor. Next, I moved the papers around like pieces in a puzzle until they were in an order that made sense. I numbered each sheet of paper, using a stick-on Post-it. Then I sat down and wrote a cover letter to go with the package of material. Next, I saw myself at the copy center photocopying the package of material I had put together.

The next morning when I awoke, I remembered every detail of what I had done in my dream. That day, I got busy pulling out all the boxes of material I had put away. I put together the appropriate material that I retrieved from the storage boxes and then wrote a cover letter explaining, in general terms, how everything should be used. Then I was ready to head for the local copy shop.

While at the copy shop, I bought a box of large brown envelopes and a package of mailing labels. After completing several dozen sets of copies and checking to make sure that everything would fit, I headed home.

Each time a new person contacted me, I would explain that there was too much information to discuss over the phone but that I would mail an information package containing a general overview of the program I had put together. It was my hope that each person would be able to duplicate the program I had used and adjust it to his or her own particular needs and situation.

Most of the people who contacted me and whom I mailed packages of information to never contacted me again. I don't know if they tried it on their own or just did not accept the alternative approach.

Some people did call after receiving the information package and asked specific questions about how I used the different therapies. I would try to help them set up their own individualized healing program over the telephone. Sometimes this process would require a number of conversations during the first couple of weeks.

Other people who called wanted me to come to their homes and teach them how to do the meditation, visualization, and guided imagery, as well as check their use of the wet cell. They also wanted to make sure that they were maintaining the equipment properly. Mostly, they wanted me to teach them how to develop and use a personalized healing program that would fit their specific needs.

It was at this point in time that I realized they expected more from me than I was equipped to give. I had no training in these alternative therapies that I had used to reverse my symptoms. I had no experience in teaching others how to do what I had taught myself. It was time for me to get my feet on the ground. There were a lot of questions that I had to ask myself: Should I be taking on this kind of serious responsibility? Can I really make a difference in the lives of some of these people? Suppose

I could teach someone to do what I did and they got better! Maybe I would be able to help some ALS people and their families deal more effectively with their illness, allowing them to live a longer and better quality life. Maybe it wouldn't work for other people.

I remembered back to when I was in the same situation these people now found themselves in and how I had felt. Somebody had to quiet their fear, raise their spirits, and help them and their families deal with what was happening in their lives.

The doctors had made it clear that there wasn't anything they could offer. I could remember the feeling of despair and of powerlessness. That lost feeling only made a bad situation worse. I meditated and prayed, seeking answers to these important questions that had become a great concern to me.

After several days of having long conversations with myself and with God, I experienced that old but familiar feeling of a presence all around me. I was overcome by a warm excitement, almost like a rush of energy swirling within me. I was made aware, I had a "knowing," and the answers came to me rapidly. Yes, I should be ministering to these people who are crying out for help. Yes, I can make a difference in some of their lives and the lives of their families.

There were also specific instructions about things I needed to do to prepare for the task ahead of me. I needed to study and learn about all the therapies that I would teach. I could not just say I did it. I had to know how to teach each person how to do it for himself or herself, because in doing for one's self there is hope of achievement. I should not attempt to do anything for them, other than give them the tools to help themselves and the light of hope. I know only too well from personal experience that if someone has no hope, then he or she has nothing.

As I started to study and educate myself, I participated in a number of workshops and training sessions regarding meditation, visualization, and guided imagery, as well as the importance of attitude and being a loving and caring person. I studied a number of different massage techniques, stress reduction and management, biofeedback, hypnotherapy, pain management, and preventive medicine.

Fortunately, I had been introduced to one of the leading organizations in the world dedicated to fostering education for the benefit of humankind—the A.R.E.

A nonprofit organization, the A.R.E. has headquarters in Virginia Beach, Virginia, ten regional areas located throughout the U.S., and eleven regional offices located throughout Canada. International facilities are located in Australia, Belgium, Colombia, Costa Rica, the Czech Republic, Denmark, Ecuador, England-U.K., France, Germany, Greece, Holland, Ireland, Japan, Mexico, New Zealand, the Philippines, Poland, South Africa, Sweden, and Trinidad.

The A.R.E. has continuing educational programs, workshops, and seminars presented throughout the year at the headquarters campus in Virginia Beach. The campus consists of the Cayce/Reilly School of Massotherapy, the Edgar Cayce library (housing more than 14,000 readings), a modern conference center, a beautiful meditation garden, and the A.R.E. Press complex. Study Groups and other educational programs are offered in the regional areas throughout the world. There is also the A.R.E. Youth and Family Camp located in the beautiful Blue Ridge Mountains. Scheduled programs operate there May through August.

During the time that I was studying and learning all the material necessary to acquire the skills I needed, I contacted Bruce Baar regarding the wet cell unit and explained what I was doing and asked if he would answer any of the technical questions that people might raise about the wet cell unit. He agreed to assist in any way that he could. Both he and his wife, Kathy, have helped me many times, and I am sure that I have failed to thank them sufficiently for their encouragement and moral support. So, I say to you both, I love you and I thank you!

The Presbyterian Hospital, located in Charlotte, North Carolina, had opened the Center for Mind-Body Health, where doctors could refer patients who were experiencing serious illnesses. At the Center, patients could learn to use their minds to help regulate their bodies, regarding stress and healing.

The Center offered an extensive eight-week program incorporating the components of healing, such as mindfulness, moment-to-moment awareness, self-regulation, self-directed change, general relaxation, and regulating of the body and mind, as well as activities of the mind, such as mind-talk, thoughts, feelings, images, sensations, mindfulness, attention, concentration, and meditation. Other programs included "How Caring Relationships Aid the Heart and Soul" and "Nutritional Care Plan," taught by a clinical dietitian and nutritionist.

This kind of program was exactly what I had been searching for. What I learned validated the therapies that I had used to help reverse my illness, as well as gave me the medical theories and explanations that supported the reason why these therapies worked.

Our study guide during the program was a remarkable book entitled *Full Catastrophe Living—Using the Wisdom of Your Body and Mind to Face Stress, Pain, and Illness.* The author is Jon Kabat-Zinn, Ph.D., founder and director of the Stress Reduction Clinic at the University of Massachusetts Medical Center and associate professor of medicine in the Division of Preventive and Behavioral medicine at the University of Massachusetts Medical School.

One of the chapters that I found most interesting was Chapter 15, "Mind and Body: Evidence That Beliefs, Attitudes, Thoughts, and Emotions Can Harm or Heal." Optimism and pessimism—to a great extent—control how we perceive the things that happen around us and to us. Optimism is a positive mental thought process. When bad things happen to people who are optimists, they generally focus on what happens, rather than fantasizing and making a bad situation worse. And they tend to not blame themselves for the bad event.

During a bad event, a pessimist most likely would say something like this: "If there weren't bad luck, I wouldn't have any luck at all!" They have a tendency to feel that they attract bad events to themselves. Pessimists are at significantly higher risk of becoming depressed and can show negative immune system changes.

On the other hand, an optimist can produce good body chemistry during a bad event just by the manner in which he or she perceives the event. Confidence in one's ability to overcome bad events influences a person's ability to accomplish what he or she believes. Dr. Albert Bandura and his colleagues at Stanford University Medical School have shown that "a strong sense of self-efficacy is the best and most consistent predictor of positive health outcomes in many different medical situations."

Self-esteem—believing in one's self and feeling that one deserves to recover from an illness—is a positive self-healing influence that becomes self-perpetuating. A positive attitude can be developed by mindfulness. A person needs to be aware when he or she is experiencing negative thoughts or negative mind-talk and then replace those negative thoughts with positive ones. As one becomes proficient at this process, his or her attitude will become more positive. It's a mental learning exercise that changes the direction of mind-talk, enabling a person to improve his or her attitude.

One's emotions should not be suppressed, and the manner in which one deals with emotions is an important factor involved in healing. Anger, hostility, cynicism, and fear must be replaced with understanding, caring, hope, and love.

Social factors also can play a major role in health. Jon Kabat-Zinn writes: "It has long been known, for instance, that, statistically speaking, people who are socially isolated tend to be less healthy psychologically and physically, and more likely to die prematurely than people who have extensive social relationships." The insights of Kabat-Zinn and the way in which he expressed his knowledge created a profound learning experience for me and offered me new options to use when working with others.

I am grateful to Dr. Joe Parisi, director of psychology and behavioral medicine at Presbyterian Hospital for making the program available to me.

Something that I came across while reading one of the many books that are now part of my reference library was an interesting scale used as a predictor of potential illness. Using this scale, I evaluated my life prior to the onset of my illness. The results were fascinating because, at least in my situation, they were right on target.

The Holmes-Rahe Social Readjustment Scale was developed by physicians Thomas Holmes and Richard Rahe to reflect the disruptive effects of certain changes in a person's life. Dr. Holmes and Dr. Rahe suggested that a score exceeding 300 in one year indicated an 80 percent probability of developing a serious illness. Because everyone reacts to change differently, the scale is best used as a general measure of the relative stress from life events.

(This scale was developed in 1960. Thirty-seven years have passed and the LIFE EVENTS and MEAN VALUE are not representative of today. But the scale can be used as a guide.)

RANK	LIFE EVENT	MEAN VALUE
1	Death of spouse	100
2	Divorce	73
3	Marital separation	65
4	Jail term	63
5	Death of close family member	63
6	Personal injury or illness	53
7	Marriage	50
8	Fired at work	47
9	Marital reconciliation	45
10	Retirement	45
11	Change in health of family member	44
12	Pregnancy	40
13	Sex difficulties	39
14	Gain of a new family member	39
15	Business readjustment	39
16	Change in financial state	38
17	Death of a close friend	37
18	Change to different line of work	36
19	Change in number of arguments with spouse	35
20	Mortgage over $10,000	31
21	Foreclosure of mortgage or loan	30
22	Change in responsibilities at work	29
23	Son or daughter leaving home	29
24	Trouble with in-laws	29
25	Outstanding personal achievement	28
26	Wife begins or stops work	28
27	Beginning or ending school	26
28	Change in living conditions	26

29	Revision of personal habits	24
30	Trouble with boss	23
31	Change in work hours or conditions	20
32	Change in residence	20
33	Change in school	20
34	Change in recreation	19
35	Change in church activities	19
36	Change in social activities	18
37	Mortgage or loan less than $10,000	17
38	Change in sleeping habits	16
39	Change in number of family get-togethers	15
40	Change in eating habits	15
41	Vacation	13
42	Christmas	12
43	Minor violation of the law	11

As you can see, not all stressful events fall into a category of being bad or negative experiences. And as I have learned, it's not really the event that does the damage—rather it's the way one perceives the event and how the person responds to that perception that causes health-related problems.

During this educational period that I was going through, I also read numerous articles, research papers, and books that related to the mind-body approach to healing. I studied the successful programs developed and used by Dr. O. Carl Simonton, M.D., and Stephanie Matthews-Simonton, as well as the E-Cap program developed by Bernie Siegel, M.D. (more about these later).

While continuing my educational research, I came across an interesting article about the Monroe Institute. What I read was exciting and helped to reinforce my belief in the power of the mind to regulate and help heal the physical body.

The Monroe Institute is a nonprofit educational and

research organization. The legacy of the Institute began in 1956, when Robert Monroe established a research and development division of his corporation to study the feasibility of learning during sleep. From the achievements of this early research, Monroe and his group began to focus on various methods to induce specific states of consciousness in their laboratory. Their efforts gradually produced significant results that attracted professionals from other disciplines. With this increased interest, Mr. Monroe developed methods and techniques that supported hemispheric synchronization. Today this process is known as Hemi-Sync. Hemispheric synchronization is when patterns of sound are used to create simultaneously an identical wave form in both brain hemispheres. Hemi-Sync has been awarded three patents and is the subject of numerous articles found in a variety of publications. Hemi-Sync is widely used in a variety of professional applications in the form of a state-of-the-art auditory-guidance technology produced on Hemi-Sync audiocassettes and CDs.

In 1974, the Monroe Institute evolved from the original research group and began conducting learning seminars in self-control of human consciousness. These seminars were held at various sites, both in the U.S. and abroad, until 1979 when a facility was built in the Blue Ridge Mountains of Virginia.

As I read about one of the many residential programs offered at the Institute, the six-day intensive Gateway Voyage program, I had one of my "knowing" experiences. This particular program is an adventure into self-discovery and provides participants with tools for the development and exploration of human consciousness, expansion of one's awareness, and enhancement of physical, mental, and emotional processes.

That is exactly what I had been experiencing, but I didn't understand how to bring it all together or how to use this awareness to help myself, as well as other people.

I contacted Bob Monroe, explaining about my personal experience with illness and how I had been called to help others. His response was caring and very exciting for me. He invited me to come to the Monroe Institute as his guest and take part in the Gateway Voyage program. I will forever be grateful to Bob Monroe for a most profound learning experience that has changed my life in many positive ways and has also given me an additional healing tool to use, in the form of the Hemi-Sync tapes.

The prayer that I had been using regularly asking for guidance and direction to those people, places, and things that could help me to help myself certainly was answered on a consistent basis. None of these good things that were flowing into my life was accidental or good luck. Each was a result of my growing as a complete human being and the realization that, in fact, we are all first and foremost spiritual beings who are living a human earthly experience.

I was ready to take on the challenge that had been presented to me. I felt strong and confident that I was doing what I was supposed to be doing with my life—helping and caring about all of humanity, especially those who asked for my help.

13

I started responding to those people who asked me to come to their homes and work with them and their families. I made it clear that I did not charge any fee for my help, that I was volunteering my time and services. Of course, I couldn't afford to pay for transportation, lodging, and food while traveling to help people. In fact, the financial burden of making up the information packages, purchasing the mailing envelopes and labels, plus postage, and returning phone calls was more than we could afford, but somehow each month Wendy would adjust our budget and make it work.

It was time to change the cover letter that I sent out with each information package. The packages had grown in size as I came across new information that I knew would be helpful. I added to the cover letter a statement explaining that I was more than happy and willing to volunteer my time to help people wherever they lived but they would have to be responsible for providing my transportation, lodging, and meals.

I had so many requests to travel to different states that an unforeseen problem developed. Because air fares were much cheaper if I stayed over a Saturday night, everyone scheduled flights that required me to be away from home over the weekend, and the weekend was the only time that Wendy, Amanda, and I had to do things together as a family. Sometimes I was away for three or four weekends in a row

It was necessary to make a change regarding when I would be available to work with people. It was a hard decision to make, because it meant that the expense of the air fare would be more costly. But my time with my family was very important to me and my well-being. It didn't make sense to have fought so hard to live and then waste any of the time that I could spend with Wendy and Amanda, as well as with my older children.

As time went by, there was a recurring problem that surfaced. What role should religion play in the program that I taught? I was dealing with Christians from different denominations, Jews, Muslims, Hindus, and some people who didn't identify with any particular religion.

The most difficult situation to deal with was when a patient would say, "I've made a deal with God. If He will heal me, then I will dedicate the rest of my life to doing His work here on earth." Then they would say, "My disease is in God's hands now!" This was a very delicate situation to deal with, and I would try to work around it. I didn't want to offend patients or any of their family members, but I was very uncomfortable with the idea that people thought they could make this kind of deal or, for that matter, any kind of deal with their Creator. First of all, this attitude went against one of the fundamental beliefs in my program. I believed, and tried to teach, that everyone had to be responsible for the decision-making process about his or her own wellness.

Being responsible and making choices allowed patients to have some control over their lives, instead of letting the doctors and other people make all the decisions for them. Responsibility empowered the patients, gave them a renewed feeling of self-worth as intelligent, thinking human beings, and created a positive aspect to a situation that had been filled only with negatives and despair.

Being at home over the weekends with my family gave me a chance to turn my thoughts to lighter problems: What needed to be done in the yard? Is it time to have the oil changed in the car? Should we take a picnic lunch and drive to some pretty park or maybe out to the lake and enjoy all the wonders that nature had to offer?

Also, I had a chance to renew my energy. I love Wendy very much, and just being near her made me feel good. Amanda brought great joy into my life. She really is a great kid, and it is very important to me to see her happy and enjoying life. Wendy and I both tried in whatever way we could to see that Amanda had a chance to experience as many of the good and positive things as life had to offer.

Late one Sunday evening, I was reading, Amanda was already in bed, and Wendy was ready to call it quits for the day. I was reading an interesting article and wasn't feeling very sleepy. Wendy came over to where I was sitting. "I think that I'll stay up for a while longer and finish this article," I said. Wendy smiled and said, "Don't stay up too late, dear. Remember you have a busy day tomorrow." She leaned over and we kissed. We both told each other good night and said, "I love you!"

The article had been very interesting, but I was glad to be finished, because I was starting to feel sleepy myself and was ready for bed. Just at that moment, the problem regarding how to deal with religion in teaching my program popped into my mind. This was a problem that had to be resolved very soon because in many situations it was interfering with how effective the program could be.

I usually said prayers after I was in bed, but I decided to ask for guidance while I was still sitting in the family room. I prayed that my awareness be raised and that I be guided to an answer regarding the recurring problem of how to deal with religion as part of the program I was teaching. I went to bed, said my usual prayers, and got a good night's sleep.

The next day, as I sorted through our mail, a gray envelope from Harvard Medical School caught my eye. I checked to make sure it was addressed to me. Yes, there was my name, right on the front, along with the words *spirituality and healing.* I proceeded to read from top to bottom as follows: Harvard Medical School Department of Continuing Education and The Mind/Body Medical Institute, Deaconess Hospital, present *Spirituality and Healing in Medicine* under the Direction of Herbert Benson, M.D.

As I turned to the second page, I realized this was an invitation for me to participate in a course being offered in conjunction with Harvard Medical School. My first thought was one of confusion. Where did they get my name and why had I received this invitation?

I had read several of Dr. Benson's books and knew he was at the forefront of leading research that had, through the use of empirical scientific studies, proven the ability of the mind to help control functions in the body. Dr. Benson and his colleagues from Harvard had studied and documented in Tibet, more than twenty-five years ago, the ability of Buddhist monks to control many of their physical bodily functions, including raising their body temperatures dramatically by means of their thought processes.

I continued to read: "The objective of this course is to explore the relationship between spirituality and healing in medicine and to give perspectives from world religions. The physiological, neurological, and psychological effects of healing resulting from spirituality also will be discussed." The literature went on to list the faculty who would be involved in teaching the course, under the direction of Dr. Benson.

Next was listed the course schedule, which consisted of three days of very intensive subject matter: "This course is to provide participants with an understanding of • The relationship between spirituality and healing from the perspective of major world religions • The scientific evidence for the effects of spirituality on healing • The physiologic and neurologic effects of healing resulting from spirituality • The relationship amongst healing, spirituality, and mind/body effects."

As I sat there and read over the material again, I became aware of what this piece of mail represented. Once again, a specific prayer of mine had been answered. This course would teach me how to deal with the recurring problem that I was having with some of the people with whom I worked—the very same problem that I had prayed about the night before! A feeling of gratitude came over me, and I said a prayer of thanks to my Creator.

My next thought concerned how I was going to be involved in this course. What sort of plan was I going to be able to come up with so that I could take advantage of this amazing opportunity? I had to determine how I was going to finance my trip to Boston, make financial arrangements for a place to stay, cover the cost of my meals for the three days, and pay for the cost of the course. There wasn't any extra money in our personal budget to pay for this course or the trip.

I knew that I had received that invitation from Harvard as an answer to my prayer, so there must be avenues open to me to accomplish what needed to be done. I spent three days meditating and praying for guidance and direction that would give me the answer to how I could find the resources that would allow me to take advantage of this unique gift.

On the third night, I was feeling very frustrated and tired, so I decided to go to bed early. I said my usual prayers of thanks and prayed for my family members and others. But my last prayer that night was, once again, to ask for guidance and direction as to how I could attend the course.

When I awoke the next morning, I had the answers that I had prayed for! I had experienced an extremely vivid dream, and I knew exactly what I needed to do. Following the dream exactly, I faxed copies of the stories that had been written about me to Dr. Benson, along with a request for the lowest possible tuition that would allow me to attend the course. Then I called Dr. Benson on the telephone to verify that he had personally received my fax. He was very gracious and worked out a special tuition for me. He had read over my material and was looking forward to meeting me.

Next, I called an ALS family who lived in Boston. I had been working with them by telephone, and after I explained the situation, they were more than happy to provide me with a place to stay and meals for three days. I was concerned about the logistics of using buses and taxis in a large city like Boston, but that problem solved itself. The family I was to stay with lived within three blocks of where the course was being offered! My love, as well as my gratitude, go to Michael G., Paulina I., and Sophia M. for their hospitality and friendship.

In addition, I talked to several physician friends who, in my dream, were willing to help financially. I explained in detail about the course and the reason I felt it was important for me to attend. Of course, I didn't tell them about my dream; though they were friends, I wasn't sure how they would respond to something that unusual. Fortunately, they agreed with my reasons for wanting to attend the course and gave me the funds needed to purchase my airline ticket. The details from my dream had become reality. There are no words to describe the impact that these glorious events have had on my life.

The course was exactly what I needed. It gave me an additional perspective to integrate into my healing program, but, more important, it helped me understand the difference between religion and spirituality. Spirituality can take many forms, such as those incorporated in the Standards of Practice of the Association of Holistic Nursing: "values, meaning and purpose; a turning inward to the human traits of honesty, love, caring, wisdom, imagination, and compassion; the existence of a quality of a higher authority, guiding spirit, or transcending that is mystical; a flowing dynamic balance that allows and creates healing of body, mind, spirit; sometimes involves organized religion."

Rather than spending time discussing the particular religious beliefs of an individual or his or her family members, which really were none of my business, I could now use spirituality as the vehicle necessary to include, in my program, the universal healing power of love that is available to every human being from his or her Creator.

My adventure in Boston was everything that I had prayed for and more. Even though we started early in the morning and worked through to late afternoon, the three days passed quickly. I met Dr. Benson and had a chance to spend some time speaking with him on the first and second days.

There were a number of other informative and interesting people whom I had a chance to spend time with, discussing some of the research involving mind-body healing, which had been in progress for more than twenty-five years at Harvard University, as well as the School of Medicine there. The research established that the mind could produce a specific set of physiological changes in the body. These changes are the opposite of those induced by stress and are effective therapy in a number of diseases.

I knew that spirituality had been an intricate part of my healing process, but I thought that was because I had been far removed from a spiritual life before my illness. Now I realize that everyone needs to renew and nurture a spiritual life, not only to heal but to continue to grow as a human being or, more precisely, to realize that we are truly spiritual beings from the time of our creation and that our human form seems to be that part we are most aware of during our earthly life.

I believe that it is imperative for us all to raise our awareness during our earthly life, in order to include more understanding of our spiritual foundation. Dr. Benson wrote that spirituality is "expressed as experiencing the presence, of a power, a force, an energy, or what is perceived of as God and this presence is close to the person."

There were many exciting and thought-provoking experiences that took place during my time in Boston, and I would like to share some excerpts from an impassioned speech given by George Gallup, Jr., that raised and expanded the level of my awareness considerably:

"If the focus of the twentieth century has been on outer space, the focus of the twenty-first century may well be on inner space. Many believe we are entering a new era of discovery—not of the world around us but of the world within.

"Certainly the times are more hospitable to the bringing of science and religion together than they were at the beginning of the century. And exciting empirical evidence has steadily mounted in recent decades to reveal the extraordinary depth and variety of the spiritual life—its relationship to emotional, psychological, and physical health—and its implications for elevating societies around the globe.

"The disappointment of the external world—the headlong pursuit of hedonism and materialism and the callous disregard of people for each other—all have driven people to look within themselves for ways to understand and deal with life. There are clear signs that people in all societies have an intense hunger for healing of mind, body, and soul.

"For the first time in history, a majority of Americans are dying, not from unconquered diseases but from self-inflicted problems such as smoking, alcohol abuse, lack of exercise, use of illegal drugs, and poor diet.

"Why do Americans appear to be succumbing to such self-destructive tendencies? The root cause may be spiritual malaise—feelings of emptiness and disconnectedness from God and one's fellow human beings, even a sense of hopelessness about the state of the nation and the world.

"Happily, surveys document two countertrends that may in the long run be profoundly healing both for individuals and for society: namely, a search for spiritual moorings and meaning in life and, related to this, a search for deeper and more meaningful relationships with other people.

"Evidence is growing every day to reveal the extraordinary impact of spirituality on humans, leading to healing, as well as to dramatically changed lifestyles. The implications for improved relationships among groups and nations are profound.

"Is there truly a basis for being hopeful? Many in this room who have felt the hand of God or have experienced an extraordinary 'moment of truth' have already sensed the answer in their own experiences, which often carry with them a sense of hope and peace and love."

I was profoundly moved by Mr. Gallup's words because they speak to the negative experiences that many times seem to be overwhelming in our lives. Yet they also embrace what I have come to understand to be my truth, and that is a strong sense of hope and faith in my life. And my hope and faith are fueled by the presence of my Creator, through peace of mind and unconditional love.

14

After my return from Boston, the requests for help continued to increase, and I was hearing from people who had many different types of illnesses. I was invited to speak to groups and organizations, as well as to do a series of public workshops.

People discovered that my self-healing wellness program was also beneficial for them as a preventive tool, and as a way to deal with stress and head off potential health problems.

As I tried to serve the needs of those people who continued to seek me out, I also stayed up to date with what was developing regarding motor neuron disease and the various ongoing research projects.

I continued to see my neurologist once a year, and during my annual visit with Dr. H., I was introduced to a young doctor from Puerto Rico who seemed very interested in my medical history. He conducted a physical examination very similar to the one Dr. H. performed each year. After having consulted with Dr. H. in another room, the young doctor returned along with Dr. H. to the examining room where I waited. We had an interesting discussion about ALS and the fact that there seemed to be many variations regarding onset, areas of the body that are affected, and symptoms.

It has long been my contention that there is not just one disease called ALS, but that ALS represents many variations of motor neuron disease, most of which eventually produce the same end result.

After having expressed my opinion, I expected to get dressed, set up an appointment for next year, and head for home. But this particular visit was not quite as routine as I had expected it to be. Dr. H. got my attention rather quickly when he said, "There has been a fairly recent development regarding one particular type of motor neuron disease, and a well-known specialist at the University of Pennsylvania has developed a successful test, which has been approved by the Food and Drug Administration, that can identify this specific form of motor neuron disease."

Both doctors thought I would be interested in having the test done, and they were correct. My answer was, "Yes, let's give it a try!" It would be great to finally have some specific information about what was going on inside my body!

As a result of that test, which proved to be positive in my case, I wrote an article entitled "ALS/Motor Neuron Disease—A Very Important Discovery!" I was compelled to write this article because many doctors have told ALS people all over the U.S. that I could not possibly have ALS or motor neuron disease—that I must have a tumor, pinched nerves, or an injury, perhaps due to an accident. The reasoning behind their "diagnosis" of my condition was that it is medically impossible for me to have reversed nerve damage and regained the use of muscles that had atrophied. These doctors have now been proven wrong by their own medical science!

I asked an ALS friend of mine to post the article on the Internet and on the ALS Digest [e-mail: bro@huey. met.fsu.edu (Bob Broedel)], set up to serve the worldwide ALS community. My friend Dennis graciously responded to my request. Following is the article I wrote:

ALS/Motor Neuron Disease— A Very Important Discovery!

Motor neuron disease and/or ALS can be divided into clinical subsets based on the patient's pattern of weakness, abnormalities on nerve conduction studies, and needle electromyography and serum antibodies against specific glycolipids. The following is a partial list of such subsets:

Familial ALS, which can be autosomal, or less often recessive.

Sporadic ALS
Bulbar-onset ALS
Limb-onset ALS
Clinical ALS
Classic ALS
Benign ALS
Primary lateral sclerosis
Multifocal motor neuropathy
Cervical spondylosis (produces ALS-like symptoms)
Guamanian ALS (some of these ALS cases also displayed Parkinson-dementia complex)
Spastic paraparesis
Progressive muscular atrophy
Progressive bulbar palsy
Spinal bulbar muscular atrophy
ALS-like symptoms produced by TMJ disorder
Etc.

A neurologist who has specific experience regarding ALS can distinguish some of these subsets, but many neurologists do not have the necessary experience.

Also, many of these subsets in reality are the same disease form, representing differing progressive stages.

Remember, there is no definitive test to prove the diagnosis of ALS, except perhaps at autopsy with a specific test. Generally, the diagnosis is made by trying to eliminate other neuromuscular degenerative diseases and then waiting and watching. But the longer one waits, the more evident it becomes that a singular outcome will be produced! It is similar to the beltway that encircles the city of Washington, D.C., in that one can exit onto many different roadways, each with a different name, but they all eventually lead to the same downtown area.

Regardless of which of the above titles is used, as time passes by, the determining factor will be the accumulation of worsening symptoms. Don't be negative and assume that everything you hear about ALS is necessarily true in your case! Don't concentrate your thoughts on negatives and dying; concentrate your thoughts on living each day to its fullest.

Despite what you have been told by one neurologist or two or even by an "expert," no doctor can say with any real authority how long another human being is going to live. Don't let anyone program you to self-destruct!

Some ALS patients live 10, 15, 20, 25, 35, or more years after onset of the illness. Some even recover! There are no guarantees in life about anything, but isn't it better to assume that maybe you don't have to prove the doctors right? Why not work at proving them wrong? What do you have to lose by trying?

According to research reported by the Mayo Clinic, patients with long-duration ALS have the same disease as those with short-duration ALS. Also, Mayo Clinic investigators were impressed that at autopsy the long-duration patients' neuropathologic findings were much the same as those found in patients who had died earlier in the course of their illness.

Several patients whom the Mayo Clinic diagnosed as having ALS subsequently recovered! It was the Mayo Clinic's experience that the more benign course of ALS could be differentiated readily from patients who demonstrated a number of etiologies for muscular atrophy that superficially resembled motor neuron disease.

Recently, a definitive test for one subset of ALS—motor neuron disease—has been developed and approved by the FDA. The test is for X-linked spinal bulbar muscular atrophy. Women can be carriers of this form of disease, but it mainly manifests itself in the male population.

There is some good news for those who have X-linked spinal bulbar muscular atrophy, and there is some very bad news, as well. The good news is that this form of disease generally progresses much more slowly than other forms of motor neuron disease. The bad news is that it is familial, or inherited.

As many of you already know, I was diagnosed with sporadic ALS, bulbar onset, in May 1991. I had several EMGs, blood work, muscle and nerve biopsies. My condition progressed rapidly, and I lost the use of my neck muscles and could not hold my head up. I had serious saliva problems and could no longer chew or swallow food. I was unable to drink thin liquids such as water and used Ensure (a liquid supplement) and puréed baby food, and lost thirty pounds.

After much effort on my wife's part, and my drinking four cans of Ensure Plus each day—one in between each of my puréed meals and two as an evening snack—I was able to level off my weight loss and then slowly regain most of my lost weight.

The muscles in my throat atrophied, then my upper chest, followed by my right shoulder, right arm, and hand. My strength was gone, and my stamina was very low. Next, I started falling often, and the atrophy moved into my right leg. There were some problems on my left side but to a much lesser degree.

I lost the ability to bath myself, brush my teeth, or take care of other personal needs. I was on liquid and puréed feeding for almost one year. I required nursing-aid assistance for the period of time that my wife was away from home working.

In the beginning, I read all the literature and bought into the prognosis. I was going to die, and the experience prior to my death was going to be horrible. Depression started to set in. I searched everywhere for the "magic pill," but the one experimental drug that I tried produced nothing. The mainstream drug trials that had seemed so promising were flopping, one after another. Fortunately, for me, I was forced into the position of trying some supplemental therapies that were outside of mainstream medicine.

Most of you reading this article already know the rest of my story. I was able to reverse the majority of my major symptoms. Now I spend my time working in the yard, doing volunteer work locally, and traveling around North America, doing what I can to help ALS people and their families, as well as others who have medical problems.

Recently, when I found out that there was a definitive test for X-linked spinal bulbar muscular atrophy, I decided to give it a try. My test was positive, and I sought a second opinion from two of the foremost experts in the world. Those experts are Dr. Kenneth H. Fishbeck and Dr. Henry L. Paulson of the University of Pennsylvania, Department of Neurology, Philadelphia, Pennsylvania. I met with Dr. Paulson, who examined me and discussed the disease, over the course of about one-and-a-half hours. He reconfirmed that my test was absolutely positive.

X-linked bulbar spinal muscular atrophy has the same devastating prognosis as does ALS. And the symptoms follow the same degenerative path to the same end result.

I have met only one other individual who had been confirmed with this form of motor neuron disease. It was at a workshop that I was doing in Albuquerque, New Mexico. At the end of the program, his wife maneuvered him in his wheelchair over to where I was standing. His face was grim. He said, "Your program won't work for me because my disease is inherited, and it is in every cell in my body!" It's ironic and unfortunate that I did not know, at that point in time, what I subsequently learned, because I was living proof, standing there right in front of him. But he had lost hope because he thought that his disease was different. Hope and faith are sometimes the only things we have going for us in life. Don't ever give up. It's not over until it's over!

So, I would like to say to some of those neurologists who have commented to many of my ALS friends around the country, that I could not have motor neuron disease because I was able to reverse almost every major symptom that I had: "You were wrong about my disease and should have known better than to have tried to diagnose a patient that you had never examined! Stop pushing your doom and gloom attitude onto your patients, and start practicing your healing art of good medicine!"

Doctors must learn to use the human mind with all its spiritual and biochemical healing energy, not ignore it.

I hope what I have written in this article will be taken to heart by some of the physicians who read it. I know that it will have a profound effect on the many patients and their family members who read it.

I mentioned the two specialists in Philadelphia and the fact that I had met with Dr. Paulson. He was interested in the supplementary modalities that I used and had no medical explanation for why I was able to reverse neurological symptoms that are thought to be irreversible. I gave Dr. Paulson a copy of the research paper that I wrote—and I use the term *research paper* loosely—as well as some information regarding what precipitated some of my self-healing procedures. I found Dr. Paulson to be open, honest, and sincerely interested in what he heard. But as to whether or not I will hear from him in the future, only time will tell.

The most exciting prospect, from what Dr. Fishbeck has discovered and the work he and Dr. Paulson have been exploring, is a possible breakthrough in the area of motor neuron disease, including ALS.

Now that I know that my disease is not sporadic but that it is inherited, the downside for me is the fact that I have, most likely, passed the gene for the disease onto my three daughters. This would mean that each of their sons would have a 50 percent chance of suffering from this devastating disease. Also, it means that the disease will continue to pass onto future generations.

Just when I thought that I was on top of the world, up jumps another challenge. I will face this new challenge with positive energy and the belief that anything is possible, especially if I hang in there and fight, using every possible treatment or modality, be it mainstream medicine, supplemental, or both. And of special importance is to find something that one can truly believe in.

By the way, there is still no medical explanation for why I was able to reverse those debilitating symptoms. And remember—at least 10 other people diagnosed with ALS, some of whom were in much worse condition than I was, have reversed their symptoms and are living active normal lifestyles today!

ALS along with other motor neuron diseases is a hideous illness, and many, many more people don't win than do win. But it's worth trying. After all, what do we have to lose?

Love and light to all my friends and their families,
Your friend, David

The response to my article was overwhelming! I received letters and telephone calls thanking me for sharing my experience. Still today, as I travel to work with people or do a workshop or a seminar, someone will mention the article that was posted on the Internet and tell me that it raised their awareness, as well as brought encouragement and hope into their life.

It's very difficult to describe what has taken place in my life, as a spiritual being, except to say I now understand those things that are really important, such as being healthy in mind-body-spirit, experiencing joy and happiness, and loving and being loved.

My close relationship with my Creator, though I am still working every day to become even closer, has enriched my life beyond my greatest dreams. I am able to see and understand things that, in my old life, I wasn't even aware of. I have unlocked many of the secrets that have released me from a life of being judgmental, self-centered, harsh, cynical, and in discord with my fellow humankind. I have been introduced to the glorious bounty of nature that surrounds us all. I am in tune with what I call *inner sense*, a state of awareness, a higher self.

We are not just what we observe when we stand in front of a mirror. We are all much more than just the physical being whose image we see.

I used to be confused by what is written in the Bible about God making us in His image. In my old life, I thought of God as having a head and body with arms and legs. He was an older white man who had a white beard and was wearing a flowing robe with a hood to cover the top of his head. Therefore, I attributed the statement in the Bible as representing that the physical image was the connection. It just goes to show what level of awareness I was in at that point in my life.

I now understand that the image of God that is represented in humankind is the spiritual being that cannot be seen when one looks in a mirror but lives within all of us, and we manifest our spiritual being through our thoughts and words as when we are kind, caring, and loving and when we strengthen and nurture our faith.

At the physical level, human beings are male or female, a biological necessity to continue the species, but at the spiritual level there is no separation; we are all one.

I reached my point of understanding when I realized that my faith should be in God, not in a particular religion or church. Certainly religion and houses of worship are good places to express one's faith in God. And without religion there would be no cohesive structure to bring together people who are searching for something that they know is missing in their lives. And as you will read later on, religion and attending church have some surprising health benefits.

Also, some spiritual people need the church as a base to join together so they can continue to grow. But more important is the ability to express one's faith in God by living an honest, truthful, caring, spiritual life.

It is easy to be seen in church as a spiritual person, but it is much more important that one can be seen in his or her community as a spiritual person, as evidenced by the kind of life one lives each day.

The question for me and, I am sure, for many people has been who or what is God? I do believe that there is only one God who cares through a universal love for all of creation. I have heard many names used in an effort to identify God, such as the Absolute, the Universal Mind, the Almighty, Alpha and Omega, Lord, the One, and many, many more, but I have become most comfortable thinking of God as the Creator.

Creator denotes, for me, not only who and what God is but what God has done and continues to do. In my new life, I see the Creator as an active force involved in every aspect of my daily living, from the mundane to the most complicated. I see God as an energy source available to anyone who believes, who has faith, and who honestly and earnestly tries to communicate with an openness through unconditional love.

When people get into serious trouble or develop a terminal illness, many times they will ask, "Why me, God?" But how many times, when people are happy, joyful, healthy, and reaping the bounties of life, do they stop for a moment and ask, "Why me, God?"

In my old life, I was hot and cold, on and off. Sometimes I believed, and other times I thought, "This is a myth and has no factual relevance to me and the world today." I have been blessed, my inner eyes have been opened, I no longer look outward for answers, I look within, and my understanding and awareness have been raised to a point of not just believing but *knowing* that my Creator listens when I pray. I do not know why or for what reason God directly answers my prayers, but I am thankful that God does.

Did I change because of the blessings I received? Or do I receive these wonderful blessings because I have changed from the old me to the new spiritual me? Are there still times when I have doubts? The answer is a resounding yes, but my doubts are about whether or not I am up to the task of maintaining my new life. And it is a task that one must continue to work at every waking minute of his or her existence. I have found that the more of my Creator's love that I receive, the stronger my craving grows for more. I find my relationship with my Creator to be exciting, exhilarating, and powerful yet joyful, relaxing, and contented.

It is evident to me that I have gained a personal empowerment, a life force, an inner mastery. At one time, I thought that one must look up toward the sky in search of the Divine. Now I know that to find the Divine, one must look inside one's self, because the Creator lives within us all. *Yes, we are created in the image of God!*

Many lives have been changed because of my new life and not always in the way that one may have wanted, but, more important, they were changed in a way that was needed. This brings me to what I believe is a very important point about prayer. First, what is prayer? The need for prayer is latent in all of humankind. Prayer is our way of communicating with our Creator. This communication can take many forms, starting with a very formal dialogue, such as the type of prayer that is used in church or houses of worship, to just having a simple conversation, either silently in one's mind or by using one's voice and speaking aloud.

The next question to be asked is why do we pray? And this is where things get a little confusing. Let me say I am not well versed regarding the writings in the Bible. I know that the Christian Bible consists of two main sections, one being referred to as the "Old Testament" and the other being referred to as the "New Testament," both of which have been translated, retranslated, and edited, as well as revised many times over the centuries. And I know that there are hundreds, if not thousands, of scholars and experts who will tell us the exact meaning of everything written in the Bible and that it can be interesting reading about and listening to what these experts have to say. But what I believe is more important is how the Bible speaks to the reader's soul.

It is rather interesting, when one considers how many times humankind has tried to interpret the Bible to fit its own purpose, that the laws and lessons found in the Bible are still profound. The Bible contains a complete and easy-to-understand set of instructions on how one should live life. Why is it then that we have difficulty following these easy-to-understand instructions?

I can only attempt to answer this question by saying that, for some reason, human beings have difficulty in accepting simple answers. We seem to think that if the answer isn't complicated and doesn't require an elaborate and intellectual quest to produce, then it can't be correct. So many times we just overlook the obvious.

In addition, there are many religions that don't use the Bible but have their own version of what they consider to be holy or divine writings, and certainly it isn't my job to judge other religions. Rather than spending my time worrying about what other people's religious beliefs are, I need to put my effort and time into continuing to build a closer and more personal relationship with God and living my life in a caring and loving way.

But let's get back to the question I raised: Why do we pray? Is it because we need or want something that we don't have? Do we pray because we have a problem or are in trouble? Do we pray, asking for help for a friend or a loved one? I know that I have prayed for all these reasons in the past, and I think many other people have, as well.

Here, I believe, is the most important question that we should be asking: What should our purpose for praying be? And the answer to this question has given me some insight into why I am now a good "pray-er" and why I get direct answers to my prayers. The key word is *purpose*. In my mind, there is only one purpose for communicating with our Creator through prayer, and that purpose is to build and maintain a close personal relationship.

If one's purpose for praying is merely to get something that is needed or wanted, or to get out of trouble, or to be healed or cured, or even to ask help for others, then in my experience prayers without the right purpose don't get answered, or at least we don't get the answer we want.

Just think about it. If someone whom you barely know comes to you and immediately starts asking you to give him or her something that that person needs or wants, or asks for your assistance to get him or her out of trouble, what would you think? If that happened to me, first I would think that that individual had a lot of nerve, and, secondly, I would feel as if the person were trying to use me. Of course, I know that God is loving and forgiving, but God is also wise.

Fortunately, when I started to pray in the beginning of my new life, I felt so far removed from my Creator that I was too embarrassed to ask for help from a relationship I had virtually ignored and didn't have time for. So when I started praying, after reading the passages in the Bible that Cayce had recommended, the purpose of my prayers was to get reacquainted with my Creator, to build a personal relationship, to care about God as a friend, and to request forgiveness for being shallow. After I started to rebuild my relationship, an inner sense developed. It was as if I had a focal point for my existence for the first time in my life.

In my old life, I used to ridicule people who asked questions such as, "Why am I here? What is the meaning of life? What is my purpose in life?" I was quite shallow and self-centered and just drifting through life and not doing a very good job of being a good human being, let alone having any instincts about becoming a spiritual being.

As my inner sense developed and grew stronger, I felt the presence of God around me and within me, very much as I had when I was a young boy in the children's chapel at the Cathedral. I was able to stop the self-defeating thought process that I had lived with for so many years. No longer did I allow my negative thoughts to fester and drain my energy.

As I began to throw out my old belief system of thinking that the only way to find answers to the important questions in my life was to look to other people, and as I stopped letting myself be driven by my ego, I realized that I truly had a personal relationship with my Creator. At this point in my life, I felt comfortable asking for guidance and direction and talking about my problems with God, as well as seeking answers and requesting help for my loved ones and friends.

My prayers are like talking with a close friend; I spend as much time during my prayers discussing and sharing the good and pleasant events of my life as I do seeking answers or discussing problems. And I will never forget that the true purpose of prayer is always to expand my personal relationship with my Creator.

15

I would like to share some of the modalities or tools that I used to change my life and that I teach others who are seeking something more from life than what they are presently experiencing.

There are three distinct groups of people that I work with. The first group consists of "ill" people and their family members, friends, and caregivers. The second group represents people who want to learn how to develop a wellness plan of action in their lives. They want to take a preventive approach to illness by learning how to reduce and manage stress, as well as other precursors to illness. The third group is made up of people who are seeking personal empowerment to change the direction of their lives. They are usually frustrated with their inability to live the kind of joyful, peaceful, happy, caring, and loving life that they see exists for others. In this group we participate in an exciting journey of self-discovery.

Following is a general outline of what I do when I go to

the home of an individual who is ill.

Step one: Start a deprogramming process for the patient and his or her support team. If there is no support team in place, one is developed immediately. Deprogramming is necessary due to the severe negative effect on the individual from receiving a serious or terminal diagnosis, the manner in which the diagnosis and prognosis were presented, and exposure to published material regarding the illness.

To quote Dr. Maureen Holasek, radiational oncologist: "When a physician gives a patient a time diagnosis, oftentimes the patients will program their mind and body to expire at that time. Imagery and improved mental well-being may help from the standpoint of improved immunity which is needed to help fight the disease." (More about imagery later.)

Step two: Replace the negative effect with a positive approach to the illness, thus reducing anxiety and stress to a more manageable level and creating a positive impact in terms of relaxation and improved sleep. This learning also changes one's relationship with death, whenever it may come, lessening fear and pain, making available more energy for healing, and living life more fully today and each day to come.

Most patients are looking for a cure, and they would like it to come quickly in the form of a magic pill or miraculous healing. I discourage use of the word *cure*. Instead, I encourage patients to replace the thought of a cure with the objective of buying time—time to heal, time to learn and use the program, and time for medical science to come up with some kind of new treatment.

I try to give hope to the patient and the support team. Hope can never be false if it replaces no hope. No hope creates despair, and the spirit, mind, and body of the patient can shut down at just the time they are needed the most. Hope can produce good body chemistry.

Andrew Eisen, M.D., Neuromuscular Disease Unit, Vancouver General Hospital, wrote about ALS: "There is good evidence that simply having a positive attitude about the disease extends life significantly more than any presently available medications."

Step three: Create a plan of action, establishing a realistic set of goals and giving the patient a position as team leader. The patient needs to develop a feeling of authority and control over the decision-making process regarding his or her life.

Step four: Educate the patient and support team as to the supplementary wellness tools that are available. Then teach the patient and support team how to effectively utilize these tools and incorporate them into their plan of action.

Step five: Question the patient and team members to determine how well they understand and are implementing the plan of action. Be aware of any team member who may be too aggressive, and help that person understand that the patient must be the team leader. The importance of the patient maintaining self-esteem and a reasonable degree of control over his or her life is paramount to success.

Step six: Help the patient and team members attain and, when necessary, adjust goals and expectations regarding their particular plan of action.

Some of the supplementary tools that I used and that I teach to patients and their support teams are: meditation, visualization, guided imagery, spirituality, and improved family environment, all of which have been used over the years by progressive physicians regarding every illness known to humankind. In recent years, they have become an integral part of effective healing programs, as evidenced by the number of major hospitals throughout the United States that have integrated mind-body units within the hospital environment. These modalities are the heart of my program and are introduced to the patient slowly in a precise order. They are used to enable the patient to experience, among other things, psychological self-regulation.

Many people who contact me say, "Oh, I've tried meditation and visualization but they don't work for me!" When I ask them how they have tried, they inevitably tell me that they bought a book or purchased an audio- or videotape. The problem with most books and tapes is that they are designed with a general format. An individual tries to learn the technique but does not have the proper foundation or the personal influence one receives from an instructor. People trying to learn these modalities become discouraged and start to believe that they can't master them. This is mind-body power being used in a negative manner, because when an individual says, either aloud or in his or her mind, "I can't do this!" then that person is self-programming for failure.

Following are complex tools that, when used correctly, can mean the difference between improved health or chronic pain, illness, and suffering.

Healing is believing: For more than twenty-five years, laboratories at Harvard Medical School have systematically studied the benefits of mind-body interaction. The following are excerpts from an interview conducted May 22, 1996, by Janice Mawhinney with Herbert Benson, M.D.

Dr. Benson: "You can have a powerful influence over your health if you learn how to purposefully relax your mind and body, and to use your own personal beliefs—whatever they may be—to help reduce unpleasant symptoms and enjoy good health.

"We all have patterns in our brain of the memory of what it is like to be well. We're wired for these memories. We can use our beliefs to call on the memory of wellness and bring the state forth. Our thoughts and feelings and beliefs are actually patterns of brain cells, a physical phenomenon. It's possible to use brain-cell patterns to promote health. This is a scientifically proven tool, shown in more than 200 studies to be effective. The scientific evidence is here!"

Dr. Benson has demonstrated the therapeutic value of the mind's ability to treat and heal conditions of the body from minor ailments to serious illnesses. I would personally recommend, as the basis for a sound foundation in understanding how the mind interacts with the body and how one can learn to influence his or her health, the following books written by Dr. Benson: *The Relaxation Response, The Placebo Effect, Beyond the Relaxation Response, The Mind/Body Effect,* and *The Wellness Book.*

Two of the major pioneers who developed a successful program of mind-body modalities were O. Carl Simonton, M.D., and Stephanie Matthews-Simonton back in 1976. They were so far ahead of their time, it's almost as if they had tapped into the universal consciousness of knowledge. The book they wrote, along with James Creighton, about their experiences with cancer patients has become a classic. Entitled *Getting Well Again,* it was originally intended for cancer patients, but it's relative today to any illness. Don't let the fact that it was written in 1976 put you off!

Let me share with you a summary statement from *Getting Well Again:*

- Emotions significantly influence health and recovery from disease (which certainly includes cancer). Emotions are a strong driving force in the immune system and other healing systems.
- Beliefs influence emotions and, in so doing, influence health.
- You can significantly influence your beliefs,

attitudes, and emotions, thus significantly influencing your health.

• Ways of influencing beliefs, attitudes, and emotions can be taught and learned by using a variety of accessible and existing methods.

• All of us function as physical, mental, and spiritual beings. All aspects need to be addressed in the broad context of healing, with a focus on the particular needs and predispositions of a person who is ill, and that person's family, community, and culture.

• Harmony-balance among the physical, mental, and spiritual aspects of being is central to health. This applies not only to the health of the individual's mind and body, but also to his or her relationship with self, family, friends, community, planet, and universe.

• We have inherent (genetic, instructional) tendencies and abilities that aid us in moving in the direction of health and harmony.

• These inherent abilities can be developed and implemented in meaningful ways through existing techniques and methods.

• As these inherent abilities are developed, proficiency develops, as when learning other skills. The result is greater harmony and a better quality of life, which significantly affects one's state of health.

• This learning also changes our relationship with death, whenever it may come, lessening fear and pain and freeing more energy for getting well and living life more fully today.

During my illness I read this summary statement almost every day. I wanted to incorporate what it was saying into my belief system, because I was sure if I truly believed and used this knowledge, then it could help me heal my illness.

Biofeedback has been used to train the mind to control specific physical functions, producing some amazing results. In biofeedback, individuals are trained to control involuntary bodily functions.

One is attached to a computer that measures the electrical resistance of the person's skin. As the resistance diminishes, a design on the computer screen grows smaller. Using this feedback, one learns to recognize when the mind is relaxed. By regularly practicing this same self-regulating technique, one can learn to control certain bodily functions, as well as control pain related to such conditions as migraine headaches.

The use of biofeedback has helped people learn to control their blood pressure and the secretion of digestive juices, and to regulate their body temperature. It has been used to teach victims of spinal cord injury how to regain the use of their arms and legs. Biofeedback has also enabled sufferers of incontinence to learn to control this serious problem and return to living a normal life.

A panel, comprised of medical experts in behavior, pain, sleep medicines, nursing, psychology, and neurology, meeting at the National Institutes of Health, stated that biofeedback, meditation, and hypnosis can be effective treatments for people who suffer from insomnia or persistent pain and urged wider use and acceptance of these alternative treatments. Dr Julius Richmond, professor of health policy analysis at Harvard Medical School, said, "The alternatives should be more widely used because many patients have had very little success with current drug and surgery treatments."

The foremost organization in the development, teaching, and use of biofeedback is the world-renowned Menninger Clinic with locations in Topeka, Kansas City, Phoenix, Tampa, and San Francisco.

Massage was, for many years, considered a valid medical treatment, but because of the technological revolution in medicine, it was discarded for a number of years. Fortunately, massage has once again become an important factor in good medical treatment. A recent study at the University of Miami School of Medicine supports therapeutic use of massage. Researchers found that children receiving massage were found to have lower levels of the stress hormone cortisol in their saliva.

The positive effect of music on human beings produces the release of endorphins in the brain, which control our emotions. Music can influence one's heart rate as well as the respiratory system. Music can reduce anxiety and pain during and after surgery. Music can reach deeper levels of the brain creating special states of consciousness.

My experience at the Monroe Institute and my introduction to Hemi-Sync technology has given me a very effective healing tool in the form of the Hemi-Sync tapes. Some of the tapes include verbal guidance, but Metamusic tapes are specially designed musical instrumentals consisting of wonderful compositions. I use Hemi-Sync tapes with not only the individuals who are ill but often the family members as well.

Humor can change bad body chemistry into healthy body chemistry by enhancing the production of neurotransmitters, as well as lessen the production of damaging chemical stressors within the body. Norman Cousins used humor when doctors diagnosed his illness as incurable and told him he was going to die. Cousins experimented with ways to alleviate the serious pain he was experiencing. He found that watching tapes of the television show *Candid Camera* and old Marx brothers films caused him to laugh. When he laughed for a period of five or ten minutes, something happened in his body to reduce and interrupt the pain, allowing him to sleep for several hours at a time.

He continued to use strong doses of humor along with other alternative approaches to improve his medical condition. He discovered how he could use the power of his mind to heal his body, and in a short period of time he went from an incurable, pain-suffering hospital patient back to an active person who played tennis and golf with the same vigor as before his illness.

Needless to say, his doctors were amazed. Cousins went on to write the classic bestseller *Anatomy of an Illness as Perceived by the Patient.*

Raymond Moody, Jr., M.D., wrote a book entitled *Laugh After Laugh,* in which he stated, "Over the years I have encountered a surprising number of instances in which, to all appearances, patients have laughed themselves back to health, or at least have used their sense of humor as a very positive and adaptive response to their illness."

Healthy nutrition is recognized as one of the key factors regarding good health today. The medical community has identified the correlation between poor nutrition and illness. Medical schools now require students to take comprehensive courses concerning healthy nutrition. As recently as five years ago, many medical schools barely acknowledged nutrition as being medically important.

Dr. Dean Ornish, M.D., director of the Preventive Medicine Research Institute, San Francisco, California, embarked on a revolutionary treatment plan for heart disease: good nutrition, meditation, and proper exercise. Many physicians scoffed at Dr. Ornish's plan. When it seemed to be working, these same physicians complained that the positive results would only be temporary, because the patients would not have the discipline to stick with the plan. As it turned out, not only was Dr. Ornish's plan able to reduce heart disease, but it also proved to be able to reverse heart disease!

The following is adapted from "Changing Habits," an article produced by the National Institutes of Health:

You don't have to give up the foods you like to help improve your health. Instead, choose more often the foods that may reduce your health risks.

Don't make all the changes overnight. Add more fruits and vegetables to your diet gradually over a period of several weeks. Each time you shop, choose one more low-fat dairy product in place of a product made with whole milk. Replace a product made with refined flours or processed grains, such as white bread, with one made with 100 percent whole-grain flours and whole grains, such as whole wheat or rye bread.

Add more fish to your diet. A thirty-year study of more than 1,800 men found that those who ate as little as seven ounces of fish a week had a 40 percent lower risk of fatal heart attack than those who ate no fish.

Read product labels to help choose foods high in fiber and low in fat. Food manufacturers should list calories, protein, fat, carbohydrates, vitamins, minerals, and fiber on package labels.

Plan your day's menu in advance. Use information from product labels and other sources to find the total grams of fat you plan to eat; multiply by nine (the number of calories in a gram of fat); then divide by the number of calories you will consume. The answer will equal the percentage of calories from fat. If it is more than 25 percent, you should choose more high-fiber, low-fat foods.

Choose cooking methods that add no fats to your foods: bake, steam, poach, roast, or use a microwave oven. If you broil, grill, or barbecue, protect foods from contact with smoke, flame, and extremely high temperatures. They can produce possible cancer-causing substances. Move racks or grills away from the heat source, cook more slowly, and wrap food in foil or put it in a pan before grilling or barbecuing.

Antioxidants are substances that help the human body destroy free radicals, which are damaged molecules that run rampant throughout the body, damaging and destroying the body's molecular structure. It is estimated that each cell in our body is attacked and ravaged by more than 10,000 free radicals per day . The human body generates powerful enzymes that naturally destroy free radicals, but over time free radicals damage and destroy cells faster than the body can repair or replace them. Some of the factors that significantly increase free radicals are air pollution, tobacco smoke, pesticides, solar radiation, alcohol, as well as physical and emotional stress.

Healthy individuals are adversely affected by free radical damage, so one can imagine the damage to an individual who is sick or suffering from an illness. The basic antioxidants that I began using the second month after my terminal diagnosis are vitamins C and E, and beta carotene (which converts into vitamin A in the body but also works with other natural protectors to defend cells from damage). I also use selenium, which is not an antioxidant but acts with natural enzymes to protect cells.

I also use alpha-lipoic acid. Although there have been hundreds of studies over the last forty years revealing how lipoic acid energizes our metabolism, the new excitement about this vitaminlike substance can be seen in the many recent studies focusing on how it improves the physique, combats free radicals, protects our genetic material, slows aging, and helps protect against heart disease and cancer. According to Richard A. Passwater,

Ph.D., in "Lipoic Acid: The Metabolic Antioxidant," lipoic acid "not only protects the nervous system, but also may be involved in regenerating nerves. Another function of lipoic acid is that it both interacts with its antioxidant partners—vitamin E and vitamin C—and helps to conserve them."

Amrit kalash: During my original research of antioxidants, I came across a report published in *Pharmacology, Biochemistry, and Behavior* (vol. 43, 1992). Scientists at the Ohio State University College of Medicine discovered that a two-part ancient formula called maharishi amrit kalash is 1,000 times more powerful, weight for weight, than vitamins C or E in fighting free radicals. Just one gram of amrit kalash is more effective against free radicals than 1,000 grams of vitamins C or E.

I was amazed when I read this information and wondered why I hadn't heard about this powerful antioxidant before. I telephoned Ohio State University of Medicine and, after being transferred to a number of departments, ended up speaking with Dr. Hari Sharma, director of Cancer Prevention Research. Dr. Sharma was one of the medical doctors who were involved in the research program.

We spoke for about fifteen minutes, and Dr. Sharma verified that amrit kalash is the most effective antioxidant yet discovered. He explained what a significant and important discovery this was, because when free radical damage becomes extensive, a person's body becomes increasingly vulnerable to disease. I asked Dr. Sharma if free radical damage could affect ALS. He said that all degenerative diseases can be adversely affected by excessive free radical damage.

Some weeks later, I received in the mail, as a gift, a book that Dr. Sharma had written entitled *Freedom from Disease.* After reading his book, I learned that besides being such a powerful antioxidant, amrit kalash also possesses a host of other health benefits.

I added amrit kalash to my antioxidant regimen as a healing tool to help me fight my disease. Besides the physical benefits that my body was receiving, I got a big psychological boost just knowing that I was taking something that was *this* good for me. Almost monthly there are new studies indicating the adverse effect of free radicals regarding most illnesses that I've heard of.

I continue to take my regimen of antioxidants daily and will for the rest of my life. But because of my financial situation during my illness, I could not afford to take all the antioxidants as regularly as I needed and even today find it difficult to maintain my regimen to the extent I would like.

What I have written here about the people who comprise Group One represents a general outline of the program and modalities that I used to fight my disease and that are used when I work with an individual who is ill. This is an intense program that requires dedication and discipline.

Group Two is made up of people who want to develop a wellness plan of action in their lives in order to take a preventive approach to illness, learning how to reduce and manage stress as well as other precursors of illness.

Good health is certainly much more than the absence of illness or disease. Good health equals wellness of the whole being, body-mind-spirit. The best way to prevent illness is to maintain the whole being in proper balance.

The first step is to identify those things in our lives that detract from and interfere with wellness. Did you know that medical professionals calculate that more than 80 percent of all visits to doctors' offices are related, directly or indirectly, to stress?

It's clear that our exposure to stress is relentless. It affects our life at home, at work, in school, as well as in our social environment. It affects virtually every aspect of our life. Many people think of stress as some kind of event that happens to them, but it is not the event itself that necessarily causes the stress; it is how one reacts to the event.

Some types of stress can be good; they can stimulate us to perform at peak levels. But stress can also be a killer. Stress has been identified as a major contributor to a variety of illnesses, including coronary heart diseases, cancer, respiratory problems, cirrhosis of the liver, accidental injuries, and suicide—six of the leading causes of death in the United States.

People who don't reduce or manage their stress are more susceptible to colds and flu because stress can affect the immune system. Successful use of stress management techniques can short-circuit the physical and emotional responses to stress. Learning the ability to restructure one's thoughts can reduce stress levels, as negative or positive mind-talk can determine one's level of stress.

We also must deal with spiritual stress. Stress can be a feeling of inner turmoil. Stress can be created by comparing one's self to other people who you think are successful and then trying to emulate their lives rather than living your own. One needs to establish the true symbols of success for himself or herself.

It is important not to let ego get in the way. One's ego can become the controlling power in life. Having possessions can become a way of life, especially when those possessions represent perceived monetary value and one has the need to display them like trophies for all the world to see. These types of behavior can lead to spiritual bankruptcy.

Another precursor to illness is anger. "Anger is depression's companion, not its substitute," said John Mirowsky, a professor at Ohio State University, at a meeting of the American Psychological Association. Anger can lead to anxiety and produce a completely different set of neurotransmitters, thus producing physical aches, high blood pressure, tiredness, and self-destructive behavior.

Burnout is also a precursor to illness, and time plays an important factor in burnout. One feels depleted, exhausted, worn out, fatigued, and frustrated. There never seems to be enough time to do all the things that we must do, let alone any time to do some of the pleasurable, fun activities that we would like to experience in our lives. Managing burnout requires self-awareness skills. Consider the physical, emotional, and spiritual aspects of your life. Do an inventory of how you use your time. And then write a couple of paragraphs describing how you would like to be using your time. This exercise should help raise your awareness, and most likely you will end up with five or six paragraphs describing the way you would really like to be living your life, instead of just two.

During workshop sessions, many people discover that the answer to their stress, anger, and burnout problems is also the answer to the formulation of an effective wellness program.

Helping and caring for others and involving one's self in volunteer work can be a real boost to one's wellness. If your first thought after reading this statement is, "I don't have time to do volunteer work," then you need to reexamine your priorities very closely. Stop some of the activities in your life that don't support wellness and replace them with some kind of volunteer work, even if it's only one hour per month. In a study of 2,700 individuals who performed volunteer work in their communities, researchers found that volunteers were two-and-a-half times less likely to die from all causes of disease than their uninvolved peers.

Many people attempt to solve life's problems by dealing with symptoms, rather than the underlying causes. When I help a group develop a successful wellness program, the results produce a metamorphosis of lifestyle.

Group Three represents people who are seeking personal empowerment to change the direction of their lives. They are usually frustrated with their inability to live the kind of joyful, peaceful, happy, caring, and loving life that they see exists for others.

One of the issues addressed in this group is how one can raise his or her sense of what it means to be a whole being. Part of this process involves awakening the power within, then owning that power.

Empowerment, according to *Webster's New World Dictionary*, is "to have power to authorize." Who on this earth has the power to authorize a human being to be joyful, or peaceful, or happy, or caring, or loving? And where does this power come from? The *who* is you! You are the only human being on the face of this earth who has the power to allow yourself to experience these feelings or emotions. Certainly there are people or experiences that can help or hinder, but only you can allow these emotions to happen. And where does this power come from? It comes from within you, in the form of your spirit, your will, your Higher Self. No one can lend it to you or even give it to you. You can't buy it. You can't create it, because it's already there inside you.

If we all have this wonderful power within us and we are the only ones who have the authority to use it, then what's the problem? Life should be filled with joy, peace, happiness, caring, and love! From my own personal life, and now from the life experiences of hundreds of other people, I have found that we allow barriers to place limitations on our inner power. One of the barriers is that we fail to own our power; we allow people and situations around us to subdue this all-important power.

We started out in life as very dependent, little human beings. When we were young children, we didn't know that we owned any power. So we learned to look outside of ourselves for everything. When we entered school, we were taught to respect the teacher, and we certainly learned quickly that the teachers had power. We learned that certain students in our classes had power just because they were bigger or stronger or maybe because they were the teacher's pet. We came to learn that older students in higher grades also had power.

It's reasonably fair to say that we were taught by our parents and all the other well-meaning authority figures around us to accept limitations, and as we had inner feelings and awareness of our inner power, a pecking order developed. We discovered that we could exercise our power over individuals and situations that were lower in the pecking order than we were.

During this growing period, we believed that joy, peace, happiness, care, and love, along with food, shelter, and clothing, were given to us by others, but that also meant that these things could be taken away from us, as well.

Fortunately, along the road of life, we exercised degrees of freedom and developed areas of independence. But, sadly, many human beings drag around the burden of outdated belief systems that are no longer valid for them as free, independent, intelligent, productive, adult human beings today. Therefore, many people still own some of their old beliefs, which are barriers that stop them from fully owning and exercising their inner power. The result is, in many cases, the inability to fully develop their spirit, their will, their Higher Self.

If one does not own inner power, he or she can hardly be expected to develop it or use it. Within a group setting or a specific workshop, I am able to help many people work through the barriers that subdue their inner power. I use meditation, visualization, and guided imagery, along with caring, love, and hope. But most valuable of all, for the seekers in this group, is *spirituality.*

The spirit, the will, the Higher Self must be healed as part of any physical healing. Remember: we are all spiritual beings using a physical body during our earthly life.

16

This is an appropriate point in time to discuss the validity of the alternative therapies I used for my own healing and that I make available through workshops and seminars to others who are searching for answers to serious questions. Just how prevalent is the American people's belief in alternative medical therapies? And how large a role does spirituality play in the healing process? What influence does organized religion have in the U.S.? Are we talking about a small number of people living in an isolated part of the United States? What do doctors think about alternative therapies and the use of spirituality in the healing art of medicine?

It is hoped that the answers to all of these questions, as well as many more, will become evident as one's awareness begins to absorb the vastness and the depth of the health care revolution that is taking place in our society today.

Life magazine, September 1996, displayed these

words on its front cover:

The Healing Revolution
Surgery or acupuncture—Antibiotics or herbs?
BOTH ARE BETTER

More and more M.D.s are mixing Ancient Medicine and New Science to treat everything from the common cold to heart disease.

Life magazine dedicated eleven pages, by George Howe Colt, to alternative treatments. The article began with the description of an operating room scene at the prestigious Columbia-Presbyterian Medical Center in New York City, where a triple coronary bypass operation combined traditional surgery with Therapeutic Touch, which involves the use of one's hands to consciously direct the flow of energy to the patient's body. Both the surgical team and the Therapeutic Touch practitioner worked side by side in the operating room!

Dolores Krieger, former professor of nursing at New York University, is the world's leading expert on Therapeutic Touch. Dr. Krieger teaches that there are four major effects of Therapeutic Touch: relaxation, pain reduction, accelerated healing, and alleviation of psychosomatic symptoms.

More than 40,000 registered nurses throughout the United States and Canada use Therapeutic Touch, and it has been taught in more than eighty colleges, universities, and schools of nursing in the U.S., as well as seventy-five foreign countries. Dr. Krieger has been acknowledged by the *Journal of the American Medical Association* "for demonstrating the importance of touch in medicine."

The *Life* magazine article continued: "A recent survey of family physicians found that more than half regularly prescribe alternative therapy or have tried it themselves.

"Thirty-four of this country's 125 medical schools—including Harvard, Yale, Johns Hopkins, Columbia, Indiana, University of California-Los Angeles, Emory, and others offer courses in alternative medicine.

"Even the American Medical Association, which two decades ago declared it 'unethical' for its members to associate with chiropractors, grudgingly passed a resolution last year suggesting that its 300,000 members 'become better informed regarding the practices and techniques of alternative or unconventional medicine.' "

Other information the *Life* magazine includes:

• A 1993 study found one in three Americans used alternative therapies, and it was estimated that Americans spend about fourteen billion dollars a year on this type of therapy.

• Chinese medicine is based on the belief that a life force, or qi (Chi), flows through channels in the body and can be stimulated by the insertion of needles into the skin, using some of the body's 14 channels and 360 acupuncture points.

• "Neck pain is treated with osteopathy, in which gentle manipulation is used to align the muscles, bones, and joints."

• "In a University of Maryland study of the effect of mind/body techniques on back pain, subjects learn qi gong (Chi gong), a technique of breathing and movement practiced by some eighty million people in China."

• Some insurance companies and HMOs—and the number is continuing to increase—offer coverage for a number of alternative therapies. An individual's state insurance regulatory agency or insurance company can give information about what alternative therapies are covered.

For those who may not be familiar with some of the alternative therapies, the following glossary should be helpful:

Acupuncture is a Chinese technique in which thin needles are inserted into the body and manipulated at *points* just below the surface of the skin. The points correspond to various internal organs and functions. The needle stimulation is believed to increase or decrease Chi, returning organs to a more harmonious and healthy condition. Sometimes heat is applied to the needles after insertion.

Aromatherapy is the medicinal or cosmetic use of over 300 essential oils extracted from trees, herbs, grasses, and flowers. Treatment is primarily by external application or inhalation, including compresses, body oils and lotions, baths, sprays, and the use of heated diffusers.

Ayurvedic medicine is an approach, originating in India, holding that health is a balance of the physical, emotional, and spiritual, with illness seen as a state of imbalance. Nutrition, massage, meditation, and natural medications are the central modalities applied.

Biofeedback is a method using electronic devices and computers to detect changes in muscle tension, skin temperature, sweat activity, pulse, breath, and brain waves. The feedback can be used to help self-regulate body systems or to direct body functions not normally under conscious control.

Breath work is a natural method which rapidly mobilizes the body's healing resources. Consciously directed breathing resolves stress, increases energy, and brings greater joy and balance to life and relationships.

Chelation therapy is the administering of a chelating agent intravenously under the supervision of a physician. The agents are used to bind with heavy toxic metals such as cadmium, lead, and mercury, and to excrete them from the body.

Chi is the human body's vital energy, according to Chinese philosophy. Optimally, Chi circulates freely in the body. When the body's yin and yang properties are in balance, Chi flows smoothly and there is good health. When the properties are imbalanced, Chi is excessive, deficient, or blocked, which results in illness.

Chiropractic is a modality that deals with partial joint dislocations, known as subluxations, that throw the body out of alignment and cause illness. Removal of subluxation is the key to balancing the spinal-nervous system relationship and restoring health.

Colonics refer to colon hydrotherapy, a relaxing and effective restorative procedure. A liquid solvent is introduced into the large intestine causing a washing action that removes putrefactive material and promotes regular elimination and colon health.

Guided imagery uses the power of imagination or memory to create an effective state of healing relaxation. It has been proven to boost the immune system and relieve stress. It can be used as a healing tool for the whole being, mind-body-spirit, to transport healing energy to specific locations in the body by way of mental visualizations.

Hatha Yoga is a combination of gentle stretching poses, progressive deep relaxation, focused breathing practices, and meditation. It brings about balance and centeredness.

Holistic medicine is a medical philosophy viewing the individual as an organic whole with mental, physical, emotional, and spiritual aspects that contribute to health or illness.

Hypnotherapy is a technique allowing practitioners to access the subconscious to facilitate behavioral or emotional change. It is also extremely valuable in assisting in the development of a healing guided imagery.

Massage therapy is the manipulation of soft tissue for therapeutic purposes, promoting general relaxation, improving circulation and range of motion, relieving muscle tension, and stimulating the immune and lymphatic systems.

Meditation consists of a range of methods used for expanding the boundaries of human development, raising awareness and reducing stress, involving focusing one's attention in the present moment, thus isolating one's thoughts from the past as well as the future: living in the moment.

Mindfulness is moment-to-moment awareness developed purposefully using insight and clarity to focus on what is actually occurring at the time it happens, void of any preconceptions or judgments.

Psychoneuroimmunology is the field of medical science that studies the interrelationship among the mind, the nervous and hormonal systems, and the immune system in health and in illness.

Reflexology is a type of soft tissue manipulation, in which the therapist breaks up crystal-like deposits on the feet by applying pressure around reflex points, which are related to organ function.

Reiki is a Japanese term meaning Universal Life Energy. It is a natural healing method used by trained Reiki practitioners to transfer healing energy through their hands and by thought for treatment of physical, emotional, and spiritual issues. It was rediscovered in Tibet in the 1800s and is now practiced throughout the world.

Soul recognition is identifying one's Higher Self through a sacred journey to find that part of the Divine that lives within one's being.

Therapeutic Touch is the use of one's hands to consciously direct the flow of energy to a person's body with or without actually touching the person.

Visualization is using one's memory or imagination to create mental pictures. These mental pictures can be of some actual event from one's life or can be created completely from fantasy. When one is taught properly how to visualize and practices regularly, he or she can become extremely proficient, seeing mental pictures in precise detail. When color, texture, temperature, and fragrance become part of the mental picture, visualization becomes a very powerful healing tool.

Yoga is a series of slow, gentle postures practiced, using deep concentration, to stretch parts of the body and to develop flexibility, strength, and balance.

Prayer and faith, as well, have joined the ranks of what many doctors consider to be alternative therapies. "Prayer can be as effective a vehicle for healing as many medications," says Phoenix physician Sam Benjamin, who also prescribes herbs and meditation for his patients. In fact, a growing number of physicians not only start off their day with prayer for the patients that they are going to see during their hospital rounds, but, when requested to do so, pray with their patients as well.

Prayer and faith, also, are making headlines. *Time* magazine, June 1996, devoted its front cover to this topic:

Faith and Healing
Can spirituality promote health?
Doctors are finding some surprising evidence

Time magazine devoted ten pages to "Medicine, Faith, and Healing," by Claudia Wallis. The author writes:

Twenty faith healers were recruited for a study by Dr. Elisabeth Targ, clinical director of psychosocial oncology research at California Pacific Medical Center in San Francisco. In the experiment, 20 severely ill AIDS patients were randomly selected; half were prayed for, half were not. Though Targ has not yet published her results, she describes them as sufficiently "encouraging" to warrant a larger, follow-up study with 100 AIDS patients.

A 1995 study at Dartmouth-Hitchcock Medical Center found that one of the best predictors of survival among 232 heart surgery patients was the degree to which the patients said they drew comfort and strength from religious faith. Those who did not had more than three times the death rate of those who did.

People who regularly attend religious services have been found to have lower blood pressure, less heart disease, lower rates of depression, and generally better health than those who don't attend.

Also in the *Time* magazine report was the article "Ambushed by Spirituality," by Marty Kaplan, who writes: "I got more from mind-body medicine than I bargained for. I got religion." Mr. Kaplan explains that after he graduated from Harvard University and as his life proceeded, he went through a period during which he thought that "The educated person knows that love is really about libido, that power is really about class, that judgment is really about politics, that religion is really about fantasy, that necessity is really about chance."

Mr. Kaplan developed a painful problem with tooth grinding, and, after reading about how other people with medical problems found relief using meditation, he decided to give it a try. "The spirituality of it ambushed me." He goes on to explain: "Unwittingly, I was engaging in a practice that has been at the heart of religious mysticism for millenniums."

I can certainly identify with Mr. Kaplan's experience, and research indicates that when nonreligious, nonspiritual people engage in meditation and visualization, many find spirituality just as Mr. Kaplan did. As it is said, "God works in mysterious ways."

Another part of the *Time* report is "Of the Soul," by David Van Biema, who discusses various individuals who embrace the mind-body connection and the importance of spirituality in healing. Mr. Biema tells of a physician who was introduced to the book *Quantum Healing* by his stepdaughter. It was written "by some sort of Indian spiritual healer named Deepak Chopra," the physician said. He skimmed through the book and, being unimpressed, set it aside.

Soon afterward, the physician learned that he had advanced prostrate cancer, which was considered to be inoperable. The physician thought of the book he had received from his stepdaughter and decided to read it. "The book claimed that meditation, the right diet, and a Westernized version of Hindu mysticism could prevent or even reverse disease." The physician became a dedicated "Chopramaniac" and seriously followed the teachings in the book, which required a great deal of dedication and discipline.

The physician's health improved, and the tumor disappeared. Was this a case of coincidence? Or did the physician find something in the book to believe in that had a positive effect on his illness and brought about a healing? I believe that the power of his mind, combined with a newfound sense of spirituality, brought about this wondrous healing experience.

Mr. Biema also writes about others who embrace the mind-body connection:

• Andrew Weil, M.D., a graduate of Harvard Medical School and associate director of the Division of Social Perspectives in Medicine and director of the program in integrative medicine at the University of Arizona in Tucson, where he practices natural and preventive medicine. He writes in his most recent book, *Spontaneous Healing*, "The more you experience yourself as energy, the easier it is not to identify yourself with your physical body."

This statement certainly rings true with me. When my body first started to suffer debilitating symptoms, I thought of myself as a helpless victim. But when I was able to see beyond my body or, I should say, see within my body and think of my innate healing power as energy, I developed a freedom. No longer did I feel like a helpless victim, because I believed the internal energy source could combat the physical symptoms. Visualization and guided imagery were the tools that I used to make this conversion from victim to freedom.

This internal energy source is evidenced by two examples that Dr. Weil writes about: "A man whose lungs are filled with cancer is sent home to die; six months later he appears at the doctor's office, free of tumors. A comatose young man with severe head trauma is expected never to regain consciousness; yet, not only does he awaken, but he suffers no lasting effects from his injuries."

Dr. Weil's next observation is paramount to my belief that our Creator gave us an innate healing mechanism but sometimes it requires a jolt from the mind to jumpstart the process: "We marvel at recovery of this kind, imagine it to be a miraculous fluke, the rare exception to accepted rules of prognosis and treatment. But according to a vanguard among medical practitioners, this kind of recovery is not exceptional. Rather, it is proof that the human body has an intrinsic healing system capable of spontaneous healing, and of the equally remarkable consistent repair and maintenance of itself."

- Larry Dossey, M.D., former chief of staff at a hospital in Dallas, Texas. In his book, *Healing Words*, he states: "I found an enormous body of evidence: over one hundred experiments exhibiting the criteria of good science, many conducted under stringent laboratory conditions, over half of which showed that prayer brings about significant changes in a variety of living beings."

During a television interview that I watched with much interest, Dr. Dossey said, "Because our theoretical models say prayer is impossible, scientists will not look at the evidence for prayer!" When asked about who has the talent for special healing prayer, Dr. Dossey replied, "This is a capacity and talent that is latent in every human being, and although we all have it to some degree, certainly there are people who have more of this talent than others."

• Another doctor mentioned briefly in the Biema article is Bernie Siegel, M.D., retired professor of surgery at Yale University School of Medicine. Bernie, as everyone seems to call him, is one of my favorites. During my illness, I read and listened to everything I could find that Bernie produced, and that was a lot of material. I would highly recommend *Love, Medicine, and Miracles* to anyone who cares about growing as a human being and having his or her awareness raised. Dr. Siegel is a loving, compassionate man who has had a positive effect on the lives of tens of thousands of people all around the world.

There were also headlines and articles regarding alternative therapies and faith topics reported in *Newsweek* magazine, September 16, 1996. There have been virtually hundreds of feature articles in major newspapers across the country, as well as television network programs, and even series such as *Healing and the Mind,* reported by Bill Moyers, author and television journalist, widely respected for his work at PBS and CBS News.

Virtually every day, new studies show the direct effect of psychological factors such as faith, optimism, self-image, positive mood, and social support on everything from susceptibility to the common cold to the risk of heart disease. For example, one new study revealed that married couples who are hostile in their interaction with each other experience elevated blood pressure and heart rate and show a significant reduction in immune response. The more acute the hostile interaction, the greater the negative immunological changes. Another recent study showed that divorce has nearly the same impact on heart disease as smoking one or two packs of cigarettes per day. And people who experience mild to serious stress are six times more likely to become infected with a cold virus and twice as likely to develop cold symptoms.

We are witnessing a profound transformation in medical care, a paradigm shift, as many professionals in the medical community join the American people's growing belief in alternative therapies. I am certain that any long-term solution to our ailing health care system must consider all the evidence of what really determines good health. Of special interest is the developing paradigm of spirituality in medicine. Many mind-body medical clinics, as well as behavioral medicine in general, are incorporating spirituality into practiced therapies. Health care professionals cannot ignore the beneficial results discovered by research that examines the effects of religious commitment on health care outcome.

In a review of 212 studies examining the effects of religious commitment on health care outcome, 75 percent demonstrated a positive benefit of religious commitment. Positive effects of religious commitment were found in seven of eight studies of cancer patients. And among 232 elderly patients undergoing elective open heart surgery, "deeply religious" persons and those who derived strength and comfort from religion were more likely than others to be alive six months after surgery.

The movement of incorporating spirituality into health care has been precipitated by the American public and its deep-seated religious beliefs:

94% believe in God.
85% believe that religion is "fairly" or "very" important in their lives.
77% believe the Bible is the actual or inspired word of God.

76% report that prayer is an important part of daily life.

61% believe religion can answer all or most of today's problems.

60% report that faith is the most important influence in their lives.

43% have attended worship services within the past week. (Gallup Report No. 236. *Religion in America.* The Gallup Organization, Princeton, N.J.)

Evidence continues to mount that religion and spirituality can be good medicine. Dr. Dale A. Matthews of Georgetown University, Washington, D.C., and other researchers presented the latest evidence of the influence of religious belief on health, at the annual meeting of the American Association for the Advancement of Science. Dr. Matthews said, "The research shows benefits of religion on dealing with drug abuse, alcoholism, depression, cancer, high blood pressure, and heart disease."

Preliminary results from a large study following 4,000 elderly women to see if their beliefs seem to affect their health show that "people who attend church are both physically healthier and less depressed." In the same study Dr. Harold G. Koenig of Duke University Medical Center also found that people who sit home praying alone or watching television evangelists are actually worse off than other folks.

Taking part in prayer and ritual may lower harmful stress hormones such as adrenaline. In a study conducted by cardiologist Randolph Byrd, M.D., at San Francisco General Hospital, a computer randomly divided 393 heart patients into two groups. One group was regularly prayed for by volunteers. The second was not. Neither group knew about the study, and both received the same care. The results showed that the patients who were prayed for required less medication and suffered fewer complications.

What do we really know about religion in America?

Prayer has meaning for many Americans. Virtually everyone prays, at least in some fashion, and we believe prayers are answered.

In the article *Religion in America*, George Gallup, Jr., writes (*The Public Perspective*, October/November 1995, pp. 1-8):

A clear understanding of the functioning of American society is impossible without an appreciation for the powerful religious dynamic that affects the attitude and behavior of the populace. Ironically, though this dynamic is clearly evident, social commentators frequently downplay it.

Further evidence of the power of the religious dynamic in U.S. society is seen in the fact that the importance one places on religion, and the intensity of one's faith, often have more to do with attitudes and behavior than such background characteristics as age, level of education, and political affiliation.

Nearly 500,000 churches, temples, and mosques of all shapes and sizes dot the landscape. There are no fewer than 2,000 denominations, not to mention countless independent churches and faith communities.

In the area of religious experience, some dramatic survey findings emerge. A remarkable and consistent one-third of Americans report a profound spiritual experience, either sudden or gradual, which has been life changing. These occurrences are often the focal point in faith development.

The vast majority of Americans want religious training for their children. Millions of Americans attend athletic events every year, but many more attend churches and synagogues. Professional sports events gross millions of dollars, but Christians and Jews give billions to their churches as free-will gifts.

It should come as no surprise to learn, then, that the United States is one of the most religious nations of the entire industrialized world, in terms of the level of attested religious beliefs and practices. The more highly educated a country's populace is, the less religiously committed and participating it is. The U.S. is unique in that we have at the same time a high level of religious beliefs and a high level of formal education.

Religious feelings have spurred many of the volunteers in our nation. Remarkably, one American in every two gives two or three hours of effort each week to some volunteer cause.

From churches, historically, have sprung hospitals, nursing homes, universities, public schools, child care programs, concepts of human dignity, and, above all, the concept of democracy.

Eight in ten Americans report that their religious beliefs help them to respect and assist other people, while 83 percent say they lead them to respect people of other religions. Almost as many claim that their religious beliefs and values help them to respect themselves.

One of the most remarkable aspects of America's faith is its durability. In the face of all of the dramatic social changes of the past half century—depression, war, the civil rights movement, social unrest, technological change—the religious beliefs and practices of Americans today look very much like those of the 1930s and 1940s.

Will the nation's faith communities challenge as well as comfort people? Will they be able to raise the level of religious literacy? The threat to the traditional church is that a uniformed faith that comforts only can lead to a free-flowing kind of spirituality, which could go in any direction.

There is an exciting development in this nation which merits close attention: the proliferation of small groups of many kinds that meet regularly for caring and sharing.

The growth of these groups, involving close to half the populace, and the intense searching for spiritual moorings suggest that a widespread healing process may be underway in our society.

When functioning at a deep spiritual level, small groups can be the vehicle for changing church life from the merely functional to the transformational.

Without question, the information and statistics presented in this chapter paint a clear picture regarding the depth of application of alternative therapies by the American people and the movement of a vanguard of physicians to embrace alternatives. In addition, the role that spirituality plays in the lives of patients, as well as physicians, is clearly becoming a compelling force. And religion certainly affects virtually every facet of American society.

As I began to research material and statistics in preparation for writing this book, most of the information was generally familiar to me, but I was unaware of, and very much surprised by, the powerful influence that religion has upon the vast majority of American people.

Equally interesting to me were the many outstanding and important contributions involving extended church activities, such as creation and development of colleges and universities, hospitals, day-care centers, and nursing homes, concepts of human dignity, as well as charitable programs and the fostering of volunteers.

Out of institutions and beliefs that have endured the passage of time have come the answers to many of our modern-day problems. There seems to have been an abundance of people with good ideas throughout history—people who have been deeply profound in their thinking and who could certainly be considered ahead of their time.

The following extracts from the late 1930s and early '40s are, I believe, examples of remarkable statements that were truly ahead of their time:

> For, all healing comes from the one source. And whether there is the application of foods, exercise, medicine, or even the knife—it is to bring [to] the consciousness of the forces within the body that aid in reproducing themselves—the awareness of creative or God forces. Edgar Cayce reading 2696-1

> Know that all strength, all healing of every nature is the changing of the vibrations from within—the attuning of the Divine within the living tissue of a body to Creative Energies. This alone is healing. Whether it is accomplished by the use of drugs, the knife or whatnot, it is the attuning of the atomic structure of the living cellular force to its spiritual heritage. Edgar Cayce reading 1967-1

Humankind's desire to share profound divine statements has not only encircled the planet Earth but has now reached into outer space as well. A copy of the well-known prayer "I Am There," by James Dillet Freeman, is now on the moon—carried there on the Apollo 15 voyage by astronaut James B. Irwin and left there for future space voyagers.

Just as the astronauts have started to explore outer space in search of knowledge, people who seek healing must start by exploring their inner space for answers. As I minister to people who call on me for help, sometimes

I encounter individuals who have so much turmoil within that they turn off and tune out what I am saying.

One such individual with whom I worked had a very difficult time getting by the first stage of anger and bitterness. She needed to strike out at everyone around her. She just could not come to grips with the fact that she had ALS. It was her feeling that she had been singled out and that no one else could understand what she was going through. She demanded to know why this had happened to her.

She asked a number of poignant questions, which I knew had to be addressed before there was any hope of moving ahead with her healing program. Over and over again, she would ask: "Where does this horrible illness come from? How can meditation and other mind-body teachings affect such a serious illness? How are you able to be around other people who are ill and know what to say to them and their families? What do you mean when you talk about the whole person needing to be examined and treated? Why does it matter what one's priorities are or how she decides to dress or how she chooses to use her money? How can any of these things have anything to do with my illness?"

It became obvious that she was tuning me out and not understanding the explanations that I was giving her. So I decided to write her a letter. It was important that the letter not attack her personally but instead speak in general terms.

I would like to share that letter, with the hope that its contents can answer some questions that others may have:

Dear Florence,

As time has passed by, I have become much more of an intuitive person. I have dreams that produce answers or solutions to problems that I'm wrestling with. New thoughts and ideas come to me while I'm practicing meditation, doing visualization and praying. Pictures appear that elicit a thought process that leads me in a new direction, producing a positive outcome.

I have learned how to listen to my body. I believe that our bodies are constantly communicating with our conscious mind, but we as very busy people living in a high pressure society seem to have lost our ability to recognize what our body is trying to tell us!

In my opinion, the potential for most disease or illness is latent in every human being. As each year passes, we are exposed to toxins, pollutants, improper diets, lack of proper physical exercise, separation from spirituality, and the increased pressure in our daily lives.

Our priorities become distorted, and we lose touch with reality. Achieving the highest grades in school becomes a driving force rather than the natural byproduct of learning. Looking attractive to please others rather than ourselves becomes very important. Wearing special clothing, not because it's comfortable but because it has a certain brand name displayed in an obvious location, seems necessary for some. For others, having things, whether we need them or not, becomes important, especially if they are expensive and impress other people.

Some of us become self-centered, brag about our achievements, and exaggerate our importance to impress others.

At work or in our business lives, we let our job or career cause us to neglect our families and our own well-being. We get caught up in the game of having more and being more.

Our lives become very stressful, and all this time

our body has been talking to us, we have been too involved with all the daily demands that life is making on us to listen!

At this point in our lives, we are at risk for one of those latent diseases or illnesses that I mentioned earlier. All of a sudden, that latent condition, which has been waiting to have its button pushed, gets the call!

In my opinion, most likely what triggers a disease or illness is trauma! Trauma can be caused by physical experiences or by a psychological pressure such as stress. I believe that stress is the culprit that triggers the majority of medical problems, from minor, less serious conditions to the most serious, including terminal diseases.

What kind of stress can cause a disease or illness? Could it be stress of the body? Could it be stress of our emotions? Could it be stress of our minds? Or could it be stress of our souls? The answer is yes! It could be any one of these or a combination of any of the four, including them all.

Human beings are whole, meaning body-mind-spirit is all one creation, not separate parts. If there is a problem in any area—whether it be physical, emotional, mental, or spiritual—even though the symptoms may appear as a physical problem, in reality the whole being is affected.

If the whole being is affected, then the only way to treat a medical problem that manifests itself as cancer, or heart disease, or a neurological condition, or any other illness is to examine and treat the whole being.

Unless the whole being is examined, the doctor is at a disadvantage and can only treat the physical symptoms, not the underlying cause. As most doctors know, the present system of looking at the patient as only a body just does not get the job done!

The letter got Florence's attention, and she was able to move on in her healing process.

17

As I think back to that eventful day when my body was bathed in the sun's warmth and when my mind was swirling with dreams of the wonderful adventures to come for Wendy, Amanda, and me, it's hard to comprehend what has taken place in our lives. I can remember so vividly the tall growth of dark green grass and the sound of the lawn mower engine. I can see clearly, in my mind's eye, my head flopping forward as I tried to restart the stalled lawn mower.

What a roller coaster ride life has been since that beautiful Carolina day! Out of disaster has come transformation. A true metamorphosis has taken place in respect to me as a human being! A profound awakening has grown out of the soil of despair. And the tears of facing death have become tears of joy through the all-encompassing love of God. Why me? Why me?

Some day I will have the answer, but until that day arrives, these words from the hymn "Amazing Grace" will be a constant companion as I travel the road of life: "Amazing grace! how sweet the sound, That saved a wretch like me! I once was lost, but now am found, was blind but now I see." What has happened in the past is to be learned from, and what will happen in the future will be wondrous!

Very few people are given the chance to trade in their old life, here on earth, for a new life. Each new day is a gift for me, and I will accept my gifts knowing that when they end, I will have already received so much more than I deserved.

Do I have any regrets? Yes, my old life was filled with ego-driven acts, but concerning my new life, my only regret would be if I fail to live the most caring, loving, and spiritual existence that I am capable of as one of God's creations.

Will I falter from time to time? Yes, it seems inevitable that it will happen, but it will never be a conscious, purposeful act.

No one knows what the future holds. I would like my future to be healthy, joyful, long in duration, devoted to helping others, and full of love.

Perhaps my life will continue to be blessed, or perhaps not. But whichever path is open to me, I will carry the knowledge that I was created as a spiritual being and that I shall continue to be a spiritual being when the time comes for me to discard my earthly body.

I believe that any human being who earnestly and honestly accepts the responsibility to find that part of the Divine that lives within us all can transform his or her life from what it is to what it was created to be.

My family means so very much to me that I find it more difficult each time I have to leave, either to work with someone individually or to do a workshop or a seminar. I really don't want to leave home, and when I do, I can't wait to return! Yet, I can't think of not doing what I have been called to do: "It's not enough to be good; one must be good for something!" Each new encounter raises my energy level. There are times when I can actually feel the energy transference and see the result.

I have been extremely hesitant to do what often comes to mind, and that is to participate in the laying on of hands. There have been several times when I have had no control over the occurrence; it was spontaneous. There was one time when I felt myself catapult from where I was sitting—I don't ever remember moving with such speed—to where a friend was kneeling and placing one of my hands on his head and the other on his shoulder. A tremendous energy transference took place, my hands were pulsating, and when my friend stood up, even though he was surrounded by three or four other people, his head immediately turned in my direction, and our eyes met with such penetrating force that I knew healing had taken place.

My hesitation to do what I strongly feel should be done is difficult to explain. This type of human interaction is foreign to me. I have read about people who have reportedly executed energy transference that resulted in healing experiences. I have personally met two individuals who have been tested in scientific laboratories under stringent controls and who were able to transfer energy, resulting in a specific effect on a predetermined target.

What does all this mean? I'm not sure, but it certainly causes one to ponder events that, on the surface, may seem to be so unusual that they are discarded as unreasonable. How will I handle these urges that come upon me? The answer alludes me at this point in time. It's a matter that I have sought the answer to through prayer, but it is still unresolved.

Something that is not unresolved is the source of the many wonderful people who have touched my life in significant ways. Recently, while attending the Fifteenth Annual Professional Seminar at the Monroe Institute, it was my good fortune to meet Dr. Edgar D. Mitchell, astronaut and founder of the Institute of Noetic Sciences. Dr. Mitchell's view of the universe and his profound observations regarding humankind's role in seeking and understanding the universal truths cause one to reach far within for the answers to questions concerning the far reaches of outer space and all of creation!

Dr. Mitchell, who was the sixth human being to walk on the surface of the moon, writes, "On the return trip home, gazing through 240,000 miles of space towards the stars and the planet from which I had come, I suddenly experienced the universe as intelligent, loving, harmonious." His most recent book is *The Way of the Explorer.*

My explorations of outer space, being the space around my physical being, as well as my experience regarding my inner journey, have evoked some of the same revelations experience by Dr. Mitchell—those being a view of the Creator as well as all creation as being intelligent, loving, and harmonious.

Where do I travel from this point in time? I feel that my only limitation is my imagination, so virtually there are no limits.

The thought of opening a wellness center has intrigued me for some time. It would be an educational facility, and there would be classes and workshops available encompassing an array of subjects. I envision a major program involving the reduction and management of stress, including specially designed classes for teenagers. As far as I know, there is no program that addresses stress among teenagers, yet this segment of our society is the least prepared and the most exposed.

Enhancing the overall stress reduction and management program would be state-of-the-art equipment that presently exists but is available only at a few locations in the United States.

There would also be classes in modalities such as meditation, visualization, guided imagery, biofeedback, hypnotherapy, massage, diaphragmatic breathing, aromatherapy, music therapy, and more. I would present physicians, scientists, researchers, health care professionals, nutritionists, and individuals experienced in a host of modalities as part of a continuing lecture series.

There would be an extensive in-house library consisting of material covering every aspect of wellness involving physical, emotional, and spiritual health. There are tens of thousands of people who subscribe to wellness and health newsletters in order to stay up to date on health matters. Material consistent with that found in these newsletters, regarding the most recent and timely health information, would also be available.

Imagine being able to sign up for a workshop or course that could teach a person how to be happy, how to be truly a caring person, how to raise self-esteem, how to help one's self by helping others, how to be a more spiritual person, how to defeat fear, how to become healthy and stay healthy! I know it all sounds unbelievable and too good to be true, but every "how to" mentioned, and many more, can be taught and can be learned. When a person is living a mundane, boring, frustrated, unhappy life, it is the result of one problem— the person has stopped learning, and when you stop learning, you stop growing as a human being.

We seem to have an innate need to expand our knowledge and broaden our experiences in life. When we fail to continue to grow cognitively, emotionally, and spiritually, we start to experience difficulties in our lives. These difficulties may manifest as boredom, frustration, unhappiness, a feeling of inadequacy, anxiety, the inability to function in society—all of which have the potential to lead to a physical or mental illness.

Many times the reason for divorce, the breakup of a business partnership, or the demise of a longtime friendship is because one individual stops growing, while the other person continues to seek knowledge and cultivate growth through broadening his or her experiences in life.

If you really care about someone, don't leave that person behind—help him or her to grow as well. The paths that we travel in life are not always well marked, and invariably we stumble and fall. It is during these difficult periods that we may question our commitment or that of our partner. But during these difficult times is when we may experience the most growth. With misunderstanding and indifference the copartners can grow apart from one another. But with care and love, this growth can bring unity and strength to both.

Growth is not to be feared; it is to be cherished. If the intention of two people is to share a meaningful life together and continue to learn and grow as individuals, then they become closer together as one.

It is my intention, by sharing part of my life's journey as I have described it here on these pages, to have in some way raised the reader's awareness. If this story has caused the reader to look within, if only for a moment, then I will be pleased with my effort.

If any part of what I have written here has lit the spark of hope for someone who needed something to grasp onto in life, then I am pleased.

Caring and loving and believing and having faith are interwoven fibers in the fabric of my life now. If anyone reading my thoughts has felt the desire to become more spiritual, then what I have written here has accomplished something wonderful!

It is my hope that someday in some way I shall have a chance to meet each of you—maybe at a workshop or seminar, or perhaps if my dream of a wellness center becomes a reality, you may journey to visit with me. But if our only meeting is by means of what I have written in this book, then I hope you will have considered our encounter refreshing and uplifting.

Appendix

Locating Resources

Health-related organizations, practitioners, wellness supplies—products and alternative modalities.

Air Transportation
Air Care Alliance
Free transportation for the seriously and terminally ill
1-800-269-1217

Acupuncture
American Academy of Medical Acupuncture
5820 Wilshire Boulevard, Suite 500
Los Angeles, CA 90036
213-937-5514

Biofeedback
Menniger Clinic:
Topeka, Kansas City, Phoenix, Tampa, and San Francisco
1-800-288-0317

Chiropractic
American Chiropractic Association
1-800-368-3083

Guided Imagery—Visualization—Meditation
(For information see Wellness for All, listed on p. 198
under "Workshops, Seminars, and Retreats.")

Herbs
Herb Research Foundation
1007 Pearl Street, Suite 200
Boulder, CO 80302
300-449-2265

Holistic Lifestyles
A.R.E.
The Association for Research and Enlightenment, Inc.
215 67th Street
Virginia Beach, VA 23451-2061
1-800-333-4499

The Edgar Cayce Foundation Library
The library is available to the public, offering more than
14,000 readings providing helpful insights into a wealth
of material on medicine, history, life after death, dreams,
attitudes and emotions, child-rearing, diet, psychic ability, relationships, and many other topics.

Venture Inward magazine
A. Robert Smith, editor
Published bimonthly

Published bimonthly

Holistic Medicine
American Holistic Medical Association
4101 Lake Boone Trail, Suite 201
Raleigh, NC 27607
919-787-5146

Human Consciousness
The Monroe Institute,
62 Roberts Mountain Road
Faber, VA 229838
804-361-1252 (call for free catalog)

Residential Programs:
Gateway Voyage
Guidelines
Lifeline
Heartline
Exploration 27

Hypnotherapy
National Guild of Hypnotists
P.O. Box 308
Merrimack, NH 03054-0308
603-429-9438

Debbie Atkinson, M.S.W.
Salisbury, North Carolina
704-642-0033

Massage and Healing Arts
Cayce/Reilly School of Massotherapy
215 67th Street
Virginia Beach, VA 23451
757-437-7202

Professional training in the healing arts (COMTAA-accredited program)
Health Services Department, available by appointment

Debbie Atkinson, M.S.W.
Salisbury, North Carolina
704-642-0033
Cayce/Reilly treatments and spiritually based body work

Medical Treatment Centers
Mind/Body Medical Institute, Deaconess Hospital
Boston, Massachusetts
President, Herbert Benson, M.D.
Associate Professor of Medicine
Harvard Medical School
Boston, MA 02117-0825
617-432-1525

Scottsdale Holistic Medical Group, P.A.
7350 E. Stetson Dr., Suite 204
Scottsdale, AZ 85251
602-990-1528   Fax (602) 990-3298
Gladys McGarey, M.D., M.D. (H)

Shealy Institute
1328 East Evergreen
Springfield, MO 65803
417-865-5940
Center for comprehensive health care, pain and stress management
C. Norman Shealy, M.D., Ph.D.

The Center for Mind/Body Health
Presbyterian Hospital
200 Hawthorne Lane
Charlotte, NC 28233-3549

704-384-4000

Past-Life Regression/Therapy
Debbie Atkinson, M.S.W.
Salisbury, North Carolina
704-642-0033
Psychotherapy
Debbie Atkinson, M.S.W.
Salisbury, North Carolina
704-642-0033

Reiki
Debbie Atkinson, M.S.W.
Salisbury, North Carolina
704-642-0033

Research and Education
Fetzer Institute
9292 West KL Avenue
Kalamazoo, MI 49009-9398

Meridian Institute
1849 Old Donation Parkway, Suite 1
Virginia Beach, VA 23454
757-496-6009
Researching the spirit-mind-body connection

The National Organization for Rare Disorders (NORD)
P.O. Box 823
New Fairfield, CT 06812-8923
1-800-999-6673

Sound Therapy—Awareness Enhancement
Hemi-Sync, audiotapes and CDs
Hemi-Sync, videos and publications
(For information and Hemi-Sync product catalog, see

Wellness for All, listed on p. 198 under "Workshops, Seminars, and Retreats.")

Wellness Supplies and Products
Amrit kalash—a powerful full-spectrum antioxidant
Maharishi Ayur-Ved Products
P.O. Box 49667
Colorado Springs, CO 80949-9667
1-800-255-8332

Bruce Baar
Kathy Baar
Baar Products, Inc.
P.O. Box 60
Downingtown, PA 19335
610-873-4591
9:00 a.m. to 6:00 p.m. Monday-Friday
(Free catalog upon request)
1-800-269-2502
Cayce Products
E-mail: info@baar.com
Web site: http://www.baar.com

Workshops, Seminars, and Retreats
(U.S. and Canada)

David R. Atkinson, Sr.

Wellness for All
221 McCoy Road
Salisbury, NC 28144-2221
704-636-1678
Distributor, Hemi-Sync tapes and publications
Call for free Hemi-Sync catalog

Index

About the Author

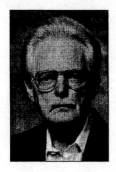

David Atkinson continues to share the knowledge he discovered in his fight against motor neuron disease. He volunteers his time and energy to non-profit organizations, conducts research, and teaches a wellness program to seriously ill patients throughout the United States, Canada, and the United Kingdom. He also lectures and conducts workshops for the general public.

DISCOVER HOW THE EDGAR CAYCE MATERIAL CAN HELP YOU!

The Association for Research and Enlightenment, Inc. (A.R.E.®), was founded in 1931 by Edgar Cayce. Its international headquarters are in Virginia Beach, Virginia, where thousands of visitors come year-round. Many more are helped and inspired by A.R.E.'s local activities in their own hometowns or by contact via mail (and now the Internet!) with A.R.E. headquarters.

People from all walks of life, all around the world, have discovered meaningful and life-transforming insights in the A.R.E. programs and materials, which focus on such areas as personal spirituality, holistic health, dreams, family life, finding your best vocation, reincarnation, ESP, meditation, and soul growth in small-group settings. Call us today at our toll-free number:

1-800-333-4499

or

Explore our electronic visitor's center on the Internet: **http://www.edgarcayce.org**

We'll be happy to tell you more about how the work of the A.R.E. can help you!

A.R.E.
215 67th Street
Virginia Beach, VA 23451-2061